PRAISE F
NONI PHE⋀

MW00378566

"I have no doubt in my mind that noni fills a nutritional niche that we all badly need to have filled. It is unique, versatile and has a beneficial effect on many levels of our well-being."

Steven Hall, M.D.
Causal Medicine Physician, Swedish Hospital

"The things I like best about noni are its potency, its fast action, its safety, and its broad therapeutic spectrum. There is nothing like it on the marketplace."

Gary Tran, D.V.M.
Director, Animal Emergency Center

"In more than 30 years of medicine, I have never witnessed a single product with such universal applicability."

William Doell, D.O.
Physician, Board of Examiners, ABCT

"Our patients have found terrific success using noni for their various conditions. We have seen low and high blood pressure normalize, high cholesterol lowered 20 points, diabetes improved to where no pills or less insulin was needed, sleep improved, smoking stopped, anxiety diminished, depression lifted, and energy and motivation increased. We could go on and on."

Susan List Mike, M.D.
John Mike, M.D.
Psychiatrists and Co-owners, Global Holistic Medical Center

"By my own experiences and my own eye-witnesses, I can say with a certainty that noni is a miracle fruit. I encourage you to read this book and discover how to get maximum benefit from this potent tropical secret that helps the body heal itself."

Mian-Ying Wang, M.D.
Researcher, UIC College of Medicine at Rockford, Dept. Biomedical Studies

THE

NONI

PHENOMENON

THE
NONI
PHENOMENON

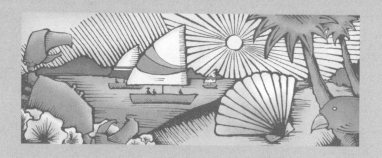

Discover the Powerful Tropical Healer that Fights Cancer, Lowers High Blood Pressure, and Relieves Chronic Pain

NEIL SOLOMON, M.D., Ph.D.
with CORD UDALL

Direct Source
Publishing

THE NONI PHENOMENON
Direct Source Publishing
500 South Geneva Road
Vineyard, Utah 84058

For questions or comments concerning noni use directed to the author, please send correspondence to the above address.

A portion of the proceeds from sales of this book will be used for further research concerning the health benefits of noni.

The information in this book is for educational purposes only and should not be used to diagnose and treat diseases. All serious health conditions should be treated by a competent health practitioner. Neither the publisher nor the author of this book in any way dispense medical advice, prescribe remedies, or assume responsibility for those who choose to treat themselves.

ISBN 1-887938-87-7

Printing number
10 9 8 7 6 5 4 3 2

PRINTED IN THE UNITED STATES OF AMERICA.

I dedicate this book to the love of my life—my dear wife, Frema, who makes me very happy. To our three special sons and their wives: Ted and Esther, Scott and Florita, and Cliff and Bernadette. And to our precious grandchildren, Scott Jr., Jacob, Bayard and Tessa Grace.

CONTENTS

Acknowledgments / 9

Introduction / 11

Chapter 1
What Is Noni? / 15

Chapter 2
Noni: Key Piece in the Big Health Puzzle / 27

Chapter 3
How Is Noni Used Today? / 39

Chapter 4
Noni's Key Components / 53

Chapter 5
Noni and Cancer / 77

Chapter 6
Noni and Diabetes / 105

Chapter 7
Noni and High Blood Pressure / 131

Chapter 8
Noni and Chronic Pain / 155

Chapter 9
Noni's Other Health Benefits / 181

Chapter 10
The Power of Noni / 223

Chapter 11
The Noni Phenomenon: What the Experts Think / 239

Chapter 12
Safe and Effective Use of Noni / 277

Endnotes / 287
Index / 291

ACKNOWLEDGMENTS

WHEN CONSIDERING THE many people who in some way contributed to the completion of this book, there are simply too many to recognize here. However, there are a select few that provided me with valuable knowledge or assistance in bringing this book to fruition.

I want to especially thank the following health professionals for sharing their knowledge of noni with me. They include Alan Bailey, Bryant Bloss, M.D., Richard T. Dicks, Frank Elaty, M.D., Scott Gerson, M.D., Steven Hall, M.D., Mona Harrison, M.D., Dr. Ralph Heinicke, Dr. Anne Hirazumi, Dr. Samuel Kolodney, Dr. Jim Marcoux, Dr. W.T. Meier, Dr. Louise Morin, Dr. Lois H. Rezler, Dr. Nelson T. Rivers, Dr. Rick T. Smith, Gary Tran, D.V.M., Mian-Ying Wang, M.D., William Doell, D.O., Dr. Joel Murphy, Dr. Joel Fuhrman, Peter Lodewich, M.D., Dr. Cliff Blumberg, Dr. Paul Dragut, Orlando Pile, M.D., Dr. Nathan Rabb, Keith Sehnert, M.D., John Mike, M.D., Susan Mike, M.D., Dr. Charles Garnier, Richard Passwater, M.D., and Haruhiko Kogo, M.D.

This book would have never seen the light of day if it hadn't been for the following visionaries who introduced noni to the world: Stephen Story, John Wadsworth, Kelly Olsen, Kim Asay, and Kerry Asay.

Next, I wish to thank Floyd and Ann Holdman, Dru and Georgette White, Gary and Ann Wilson, Del and Sylvia Williams, Mark and Jo Rose, and Ken and Mary Roland for their help in tracing the many testimonials and case histories contained in the book. I express my gratitude to Nancie J. Fleming, Priscilla Martinez, Gloria Schanely, A. Warren and Laurelle Turski, and Evelyn Kryt for helping me better appreciate the value of noni.

Additionally, there are those who provided me with many of the outstanding testimonials used in the book; these include John and

Laurie Bentley, Suzie and Caleb Kwok, Tom and Mannie Thornton, Lil Johnson, Tom Matthews, Paul and Margaret Pierce, Rob and Jaine Witty, Rob and Della Bourke, E.J. Maki and Siu-Linn Chong, Tsai Angela and Lori Chang, Carlton and Joycie Braithwaite, Sal Joan Serio, Kevin and Jenny Baadsgard, Ann Olavsson, Dr. Wen Chi Wu, Steve and Debra Gray, Marie Mehner and Jack Kelly, Jack and Stella Shelburn, Robert Fechner, John Dover, and Harold and Jesan Ledda.

Finally, many thanks are owed to Jarakae Jensen for sharing his expert scientific and research knowledge about noni; to Tom Black, Joel Neilsen, Doug McAllister, Dan Bastian, Charlotte Jacob, Mark Deterline, Erin Young, and Harry Finkelstein for their input and assistance in numerous matters; to Pamela Beckham, for her gracious willingness to provide whatever assistance was asked of her; to Lois Brown and Katie Anderson for their sharp eye and outstanding feedback; to Noni Blues singers Tommy Lyons, Mel Steeple, and Gary Romer for their inspirational songs about noni; to Colby Allen and Mac Oswald for their continued confidence and input into the project; to Frema Solomon, our agent who helped in so many different ways, and to Trent Tenney and Mark Lisonbee for their friendship and professionalism.

Of course, this book would be incomplete without the feedback from over 10,000 individuals who were willing to share their accounts of how noni brought about a positive effect in their health and well-being. Again, many thanks to all those who contributed.

Introduction

ALL MY LIFE, I have been interested in health. From my days as an undergraduate student at Ohio State University to my medical school days at Case-Western Reserve University to my clinical medical training on the celebrated Osler Medical Service of the Johns Hopkins Medical Institutions, and through 30 years of private practice, and finally now as a global health and nutrition consultant, I have lived a life intent on helping others improve their quality of life through improving their health. In more recent years, I have dedicated myself to the use of complementary medicine to bridge the gap between conventional and alternative medicine. It is for this reason that I am writing this book. Over the last three years, I have investigated the healing properties of a tropical plant, largely unknown to Americans, whose healing properties I believe can make a substantial contribution to how you and others worldwide can achieve and maintain an improved state of health. This plant goes by the popular name noni—a name that, although on first impression may sound funny or strange, may come to represent the turning point in your reaching a state of improved and sustained health.

My experience with noni has been an interesting one. Though I was formally trained as a medical doctor in the curriculums of "conventional" medicine, I have always sought spiritual intervention as to my career path; consequently, I was directed to and truly came to value so-called "alternative" or "holistic" avenues of medicine. I have always believed that good health began with sound nutritional and exercise habits and a strong spiritual base, and that trying to maintain a life free of excessive stress and emotional turmoil could certainly contribute to good health. However, I never really appreciated how intertwined the body's systems are, how feeling good does not depend just on the food we eat and the exercises we do, but also on the music we listen to, the prayers we offer, the environment we live in, whether we feel loved and appreciated by family and colleagues, and a host of other factors.

Upon being introduced to noni, my reaction was probably similar to that of many. Simply stated, I was skeptical. How could a fruit possess so many medicinal properties? Why hadn't I heard of it before? And the name—a peculiar-sounding name like noni certainly did not lend credibility to its being a legitimate therapeutic agent. But it was as if something spiritually triggered my interest. Maybe it was my friend's sincerity in the belief that noni was the "real deal." Maybe it was the mystical quality of its history—its origins in South Pacific island cultures spoke of its being used by powerful medicine men and ancient gods alike. Or maybe it was my gradually shifting philosophy from that of traditional medicine to one of holistic medicine that pushed me to investigate a little further.

So investigate I did. I talked with a few individuals who knew something of noni. I began digging into the medical literature to see what science knew about noni—where it came from, where it grew, how it has been used historically, and what studies had been completed as to its healing value. I even purchased some noni juice from my friends who were distributors for a company that recently began importing it from Tahiti. Most important of all, however, I began to question those who used it to learn what they thought of noni.

Consequently, I took my investigation to anyone who had used noni—homemakers, businessmen, factory workers, acquaintances, family members, athletes, teachers, secretaries, artists, friends, and anyone to whom they had recommended it. Soon, I had contacted several doctors and other health professionals who were either using it themselves or were recommending it to their patients. Their feedback spurred me to collect as much data as I could pertaining to how people were using noni, the success experienced with its use, as well as its side effects and safety. What I found has transformed my experience with noni into something equally impressive and rewarding.

The data I collected from the first few doctors, which was comprised of feedback from a few hundred patients, revealed some promising initial results. But my skepticism remained. Soon, the questionnaires, testimonials and case studies began pouring in. By and large, the feedback was very positive, and in some cases, almost miraculous. There were stories of dramatic recoveries from cancer, total reversal of chronic pain and fatigue, significant lessening of diabetic conditions, and many other incredible occurrences. Despite my amazement, I felt the need to talk to the doctors to make sure these weren't made up. I was assured in every instance that the accounts were real.

All said and done, I had collected data from over ten thousand case studies from more than 50 doctors and other health professionals. The findings have absolutely convinced me that noni possesses tremendous value as a medicinal agent for a wide variety of health conditions, from high blood pressure to cataracts to diabetes. This book is the result not only of my findings, but also of the efforts and research of many other professionals and the personal use of noni by tens of thousands of individuals throughout the world. Indeed, noni's use as a medicinal agent is something validated more by hundreds of years of use than by any clinical laboratory experiments. All of which, of course, begs several questions:

- What exactly is noni?
- Why haven't I heard of it?
- How does noni work?
- Can it really help me improve my health?

Hopefully, the information presented in this book will help answer these questions and ultimately lead you down the path to a significantly improved state of health and well-being.

What Is Noni?

"WHAT," YOU MAY be asking yourself, "exactly is noni?" Like you, most North Americans have never heard of it. Its physical characteristics are not overly attractive; in fact, at first glance noni may appear both undesirable and useless. But looks can be deceiving, for what noni lacks in physical beauty it certainly makes up for in nutritional and medicinal value. Increasingly, researchers are painting a picture depicting noni as a valuable and effective healing agent.

Noni: The Genus Queen

Noni, or *Morinda citrifolia*, comes from the family Rubiaceae, which is comprised of about 80 species of plants. Today, only 20 of these species have been identified as having any significant economic worth or being noteworthy in other ways. In fact, one stands out as the "queen" of the *Morinda* genus for its "conspicuous features, its multiple uses, and its supreme ability to distribute itself on seacoasts far and wide without needing human aid." This species is noni, a small tree or shrub that has been used in many cultures, including Pacific island cultures, for the last 2,000 years. The noni plant, which can grow as high as 20 feet, has large evergreen leaves, and its small white flowers sprout at various times during the year. These flowers develop into a bumpy, pitted fruit that is several inches long. Upon ripening, the yellowish-white skin of the fruit thins and turns somewhat translucent. At this point, the usually tasteless flesh becomes unpalatable and takes on an offensive odor (it has been described as having a "rotten cheese smell") that readily seeps through the fruit's skin. The fruit houses

numerous brown seeds with air sacs that permit the seeds to be buoy-
ant in water. (This physical feature has contributed to the idea that the
widespread dispersion of the plant over such a vast area is due mainly
to the ability of its seeds to float in water.) Noni has traditionally grown
in a wide range of environments, including rocky terrain, fertile low-
lands, and sandy areas. The list of areas it inhabits is impressive: it's
found in most of the island terrains of the South Pacific (including
Tahiti and Hawaii, the two areas for which it is most known), Malaysia,
Indonesia, Taiwan, the Philippines, Vietnam, India, Africa, Guam and
the West Indies (including Puerto Rico and the Virgin Islands). Noni
produces fruit nearly year-round.

Noni: Its History and Traditional Uses

By way of background, noni is believed to have arrived in Tahiti,
Hawaii and other Pacific islands at least 1,500 years ago, coming east-
ward from India and surrounding regions.[1] Who brought the plant to
these areas? Though it is not known for sure, experts believe that it
could have been immigrants from the Marquesas Islands that introduced noni to these areas. There is ample evidence to suggest that
these ancient Polynesians (as well as their descendants) used noni for
food; for cloth dye; and most importantly, for its medicinal properties.

Numerous papers, citing hundreds of references, show noni to be
an extremely popular plant among tropical cultures across the world.
In India, the fruit of the noni plant was employed for more than just
its medicinal properties. One early commentary notes that "the green
fruits are eaten by the natives in their curries." In fact, the noni plant
became so popular that it eventually was cultivated as a field crop,
used for all parts of the plant.[2]

Of course, Indian natives also used *M. citrifolia* for its fantastic therapeutic benefits: "Most of the plant is reported to possess medicinal
properties. The root is used as a cathartic and febrifuge [fever-reduc-
ing agent], and applied externally to relieve pain in gout. Leaves are
considered a tonic and febrifuge; they are used as a healing application

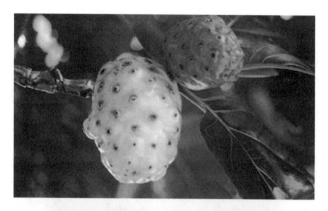

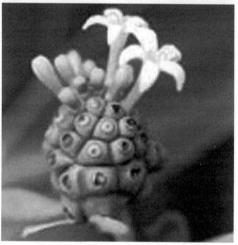

Figure 1.1: **Noni fruit from Tahiti.**

for wounds and ulcers; the juice of the leaves is externally applied for gout. Fruits are used for spongy gums, throat complaints, dysentery, leucorrhea [abnormal menstrual bleeding] and sapraemia [poisoning of the blood by bacterial putrefaction]."[3] Numerous other reports provide a detailed picture of precisely how noni has been used throughout the years: "In Fiji, the fruit is eaten either raw or cooked."[4] "Niue Islanders ate it regularly, and I have been told that the Filipinos made a jam from it, preferring the taste when it was fermented."[5] Other sources report that Australian aborigines were very fond of the fruit.[6] In Burma, the unripe fruits were cooked in curries, and the ripe fruits were consumed raw with salt. Even the seeds were roasted and eaten.[7] "[Noni fruits] are used in Nigeria in the treatment of fever, malaria, yellow fever, jaundice and dysentery."[8] Still other histories report that "The over-ripe fruit is stated to be used as an emmenagogue [encourages vomiting], and is recommended by Rumpf for dysuria [painful urination] and the fruit for diabetes. The fruit is sometimes used internally in various preparations for swollen spleen, liver diseases, beriberi, hemorrhage and coughs . . . and as a slightly laxative preparation."[9]

These statements are just a smattering of the multitude of historical references to noni and its nutritional and medicinal uses, ranging from diabetes to ulcers to arthritis.

Why Haven't I Heard of Noni?

If you have read the preceding few pages, you may be asking yourself how it is possible that, considering how widely used noni was (and is) among island cultures for its healing properties, you haven't even heard of it. That is a good question. Just as I have suggested earlier, noni has remained a relative secret in this country, waiting to be revealed and ultimately touted as a legitimate and effective natural healing agent by those not just in the alternative health fields but by the conventional medical world as well.

FIGHTING THE MEDICAL MIND-SET

There are a number of reasons why noni has remained in obscurity. But there is one reason in particular: the medical world, despite its outward appearance of being on the forefront of health advancements, is generally quite sluggish and conservative in its movements. From the time a researcher enthusiastically proclaims "Eureka!" in the laboratory, it may be years before skeptical and cautious (and many times jealous) colleagues can be convinced to surrender prior beliefs and entertain a new philosophy. Additionally, translating results into practical clinical use where people like you and me can actually benefit takes even longer.

Consider a few examples of major changes in the medical world, and the tremendous "lag" time required for the initial discoveries to be translated into practical application. In the early 1980s, an Australian doctor, Barry Marshall, a pathologist at the Royal Perth Hospital in Australia, became convinced that stomach ulcers generally were not caused by stress, as was commonly thought, but rather by a simple bacterial infection. He was so certain he had found the right bacteria that he concocted a potent mix of *H. pylori* and drank it.

Marshall got exactly what he wanted—a number of nasty peptic ulcers—and more. For almost twenty years, Dr. Marshall and his partner endured incredulity, derision and outright heckling. Ulcers caused by bacteria? Ridiculous! Everyone knows that ulcers are caused by stress and too much stomach acid.

But in the end, the two researchers won out. Today, there are virtually no remaining skeptics, and overwhelming research shows that ulcers are indeed largely brought about by an overabundance of *H. pylori* bacteria. Needless to say, there has been a one hundred and eighty degree turnaround in the manner in which ulcers are now diagnosed and treated.

Another example of a complete reversal in conventional medicine's protocol involved researcher Stanley Pruisiner, a doctor who became extremely interested in the development and treatment of various brain diseases. One of these conditions, called kuru, is a horrific disease commonly found among Fore natives in Papua, New Guinea. These natives practice what Westerners would generally consider disgusting or at least very odd: they eat the brains of their deceased tribe members. Pruisiner's research led him to believe that kuru and other rare human brain diseases were similar to neurological diseases that affect animals, such as mad cow disease.

The standard explanation during this time was that kuru was basically a neurodegenerative condition. In other words, the nerves of the brain simply broke down. Pruisiner had a different idea: he proposed that the nerves ceased to function because of an "infection" by tiny particles of protein called "prions," which lacked genetic material such as DNA. He believed that humans and animals alike could become infected by ingesting prion-contaminated tissues, such as the brains eaten by the New Guinea natives.

Pruisiner's colleagues were extremely skeptical. How could particles that weren't even alive function like live organisms? So stiff was the resistance to his theory that Pruisiner endured almost two decades of being treated as a pariah by the medical establishment. But finally, persistence paid off. Other supporting research began to filter down until finally, Dr. Pruisiner was awarded the Nobel prize for medicine in 1997.

These few examples demonstrate how various factors, including bias, skepticism, and the unwillingness to accept change, can significantly slow the process involved in bringing a promising new discovery to the public spotlight. This is particularly true for natural agents (like noni), which typically have not enjoyed much of the medical research world's spotlight due to the infatuation with pharmaceutical drugs shared by both the public and the industry alike. Unlike pharmaceutical drugs, most natural products cannot be patented. Because of this, there are extremely few companies that can afford to undergo the rigorous testing required by the FDA (which averages literally hundreds of millions of dollars) before an approval can be granted. This allows a company to make detailed medical claims as to what its product can do. Of course, there is some strict opposition to the rise of herbal and other natural products by some of those in the pharmaceutical drug and related industries. Sad to say, but business is business. Every dollar earned by a natural supplement manufacturer is many times one dollar less for the conventional drug industry. Certainly money and politics play a role in the health laws that are passed, the types of medications that are developed (and authorized by the FDA), and the overall level of care we receive from conventional doctors, hospitals and others. Of course, the industries involved in producing "natural" health supplements are also influenced by money, politics and other hidden agendas.

The point is, we as individuals have the privilege and responsibility to seek out the best of all health-promoting agents and therapies, conventional or alternative. There is good and bad in both the conventional and alternative health worlds. Our job is to investigate what we think are valid, safe and legitimate health promoting products and programs, and utilize them to our benefit.

IN LIMBO

So, noni, like many other bona fide healing agents and therapies, finds itself in a sort of "limbo," a state between initial discovery and general acceptance by not only so-called "alternative" doctors but by those in the traditional medical world as well. While those like Dr. Ralph Heinicke (who was one of the pioneering researchers of noni), and many others investigating noni's valuable health benefits may never win the Nobel prize for medicine, one day they (and all of us) can hopefully find satisfaction in knowing that noni no longer is the "secret" healer from Tahiti and beyond, but a legitimate and commonly accepted healing agent used by Americans and others across the world.

Debunking the Snake Oil Myth

Despite recent advances by the natural medicine world, there are some health professionals who still cling to the notion that any agent that is used to remedy not just one, but several health conditions, is simply a fraud, too good to be true. For decades now, the "magic bullet" theory that a specific chemical or agent fights mainly one specific disease or symptom, has been drilled into our heads. This theory is the foundation on which the development of modern synthetic pharmaceuticals has been built.

Needless to say, noni advocates find themselves in a quandary. Both the historical and contemporary use of noni suggests that it has been used for a wide array of health problems ranging from chronic arthritis and memory problems to circulatory dysfunction. It could certainly be viewed by the conventional health professional as a "snake oil" product, touted by overly passionate health nuts bent on convincing the world that the conventional medical world is against them. In fact,

I recently received an e-mail correspondence from such a doctor. In his comments, he determined that the substantial number of claimed health benefits attributed to noni constituted the "worst case of fraud" involving nutritional supplements that he had ever seen. He said that he believed noni was a product whose benefits were completely unproven and whose use could possibly even be dangerous. In reality, there is not one bit of scientific truth to substantiate his misimpression.

It is true that researchers usually identify and extract active pharmacological chemicals from plants. And natural supplements conform to standards reflecting specific proportions of those known active agents. This helps ensure that you get an active pill, but it does not totally explain why the herbal remedy, which contains additional chemicals from the plant, works the way it should, or why a crude extract from the whole plant may also work. A good example of this is hypericin, one of the main constituents of St. John's wort, an herb that has displayed powerful antidepressant properties. Initially it was widely believed that hypericin was probably the compound responsible for St. John's wort's antidepressant characteristics. However, it is now widely believed that an extract of the plant that contains a broader array of constituents than just hypericin has been determined to work even better.

Why? I believe the answer, though generally difficult to prove, is that most of a botanical's health benefits come from a synergistic effect of several diverse compounds. There are many examples of "natural" products that fit this description. Feverfew, an herb that can effectively prevent migraine headaches, is also used to relieve arthritis pain and respiratory problems because of its anti-inflammatory effects. Even more profound are the almost universal disease-fighting powers of omega-3 fatty acids, commonly found in fish and plant oils, which affect the functioning of nearly every cell of every tissue and organ, and consequently influence a wide array of disorders from brain function to cardiovascular function.

Noni falls into this category. Because of the proposed theory that noni can help the body produce a substance that helps abnormally functioning cells regain normal behavior, its benefits are many and wide ranging. As are, of course, the claims as to what it can do. And thus arises the skepticism among those like my e-mail friend as to how valuable noni may be.

With the explosion of knowledge regarding natural substances to fight disease, the "magic bullet" theory is slowly fading into the sunset. There are numerous agents that even the most staunch medical conservatives recognize as legitimate in their ability to aid the body in more than one way. Like feverfew and omega-3 fatty acids, these include antioxidants, vitamin C, specific minerals, garlic, ginseng, and others. Historical folk use, as well as modern research and use, has revealed noni to be another such agent—a medicinal botanical that can be used for disorders that affect all facets of human health.

Myth #2: "Approved" Equals "Safe"

There is one last hurdle that many Americans and others across the world must clear before they can begin to accept products like noni as a legitimate therapeutic agent. Because conventional medicines are approved for specific uses by the FDA, many believe they are thus safe and effective to use, while non-approved natural drugs may not only be useless, but also dangerous. It's a common fallacy that natural remedies are used indiscriminately for no valid reasons, whereas conventional drugs are used only for good scientific reasons after being tested and declared safe and effective.

While it's true that the FDA must approve prescription drugs for safety and efficacy before they can be marketed, once they are approved, doctors can sometimes use them for other purposes, tested or not. This is called the "off-label" use of a drug, and the practice is not uncommon. Some reports put the rate of "off-label" use of drugs as high as 50 percent. In other words, 5 of every 10 prescriptions for a specific drug are used for purposes other than those for which the drug was originally approved. This simply means that potent pharmaceuticals are actually being dispensed with no more proof as to their efficacy than exists for some natural remedies. Says my colleague Dr.

Alan Gaby, M.D., as quoted in *Natural Alternatives*, "The practice of medicine is an art rather than a science. Most of the treatments that doctors prescribe every day are no more 'proven' than the alternative methods they criticize. Accepting unproven and dangerous treatments, while rejecting safer and less expensive natural alternatives, is a bizarre double standard."

Conversely, we must realize that natural remedies aren't necessarily risk-free. Many herbal and natural supplements are potent—if not used with respect they could cause damage to the human body. In addition, there are many companies marketing natural products that make absurd and completely unsubstantiated claims as to the benefits of their products. This places both the quality of the product and the integrity of the organization in question.

So, where does this leave noni? While there surely is a need for more scientific investigation into exactly how noni functions, there is no doubt in my mind, due to thousands of years of folk use and the feedback of tens of thousands of modern-day users, that noni is not a snake oil equivalent, a fraud, or a form of quackery. On the contrary— noni is a valuable healing agent that has shown time and time again that its health benefits are many and real. No longer a secret healer from the South Pacific, noni has moved into the mainstream of today's modern health world.

Chapter Summary Points

- Noni has been used in numerous cultures throughout the world for thousands of years for its wide array of health benefits.
- Noni is still relatively new in the U.S. and other countries mainly due to the lag that occurs between discovery and acceptance of new products and therapies.
- Contrary to what some believe, noni is not a form of quackery or an overhyped fruit juice. Considering hundreds of years of folk use and current feedback from thousands of noni users, it is safe to say that noni is an effective, safe and legitimate dietary supplement with an impressive arsenal of health benefits.

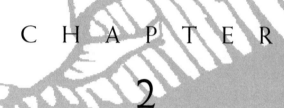

CHAPTER

2

Noni: Key Piece in the Big Health Puzzle

BECAUSE YOU ARE reading this book, chances are that you, like the majority of Americans, suffer from health problems resulting from prevalent aspects of our modern lifestyles—high-stress occupations, poor nutrition, and far too little exercise. Instead of approaching each day with vitality and an attitude to conquer the world, we typically drag ourselves through the day, feeling worn out, tired, and irritable. Sleep does little to remedy the situation, for it is fitful, intermittent, or slow in coming. Many of us cope (though usually not very well) with numerous aches, pains, sore backs, or stiff necks. We consume inordinate amounts of processed, fatty, and sugar-laden foods; we drink cup after cup of coffee, can after can of soda, and bottle after bottle of alcohol. To cure our ills, we often go from doctor to doctor, requesting a three-times-a-day pill that will lift the gloom, lose the pounds, halt the headaches, and hopefully give us a reason to smile.

Many Americans now recognize that today's health care system perhaps does not provide optimal health care, especially for chronic illnesses. All too often, the premise of the current medical establishment is to use drugs and procedures that often do not cure the problem, but merely mask its symptoms. Unfortunately, money and politics can at times be the driving force behind the health care industry. The goal of saving money, making money, and cutting costs, coupled with understaffing, exorbitant insurance rates (not to mention the tangled web of deductibles, co-pays, and non-covered items), and limitation of services all occur at the expense of the patient's health. Though most doctors start their careers with the intent of saving lives, of "making a difference," many are too quickly immersed in the political games of healthcare administrators, the daily routine of prescribing drugs, and the overwhelming task of treating too many patients with too little time.

All of this leads you and me to ask: "What can I do to achieve optimal health?" The answer, of course, is multifaceted. Now more than ever, many doctors (both traditional and alternative) are encouraging their patients to take a holistic approach to health. This includes disease prevention, dietary factors, exercise regimens, nutritional supplements, mental and emotional considerations, and a concerted effort to treat the whole person, not just the sore joints or the hacking cough.

In this holistic approach to health, nutrition plays a vital role. Be it the foods we eat or the supplements we take to complement our diet, our nutritional intake has a profound effect on our overall health. One such dietary component—noni, or *Morinda citrifolia*—has recently emerged on the health scene as a promising medicinal and dietary agent. "But," you may ask, "you just said that to achieve optimal health, we must incorporate strategies to enhance all facets of our health, and not just focus on a supposed 'miracle' food or drug." This is true—as I determined in the previous chapter, noni is not a cure-all or a "magic bullet." It may not "cure" cancer or completely eradicate other serious diseases; however, if noni supplementation is included in one's holistic health plan, then a happier and healthier life can result.

How, exactly, can noni have such a profound impact on your health? Noni can perhaps alleviate the pain and stiffness resulting from your arthritis; this, in turn, allows you to go on daily walks and an occasional hike up your favorite canyon. This increased physical activity leads to enhanced muscle tone and bone strength, which lessens the previously common back aches and decreases your risk of osteoporosis. Meanwhile, you are making more of an effort to eat better, to exercise more, and to watch less t.v. After several weeks, you notice that you have more energy throughout the day, you accomplish more at work, and you begin attending weekend religious services. Eventually, you wake one day to realize that you feel good: in fact, you feel better than you have in years.

Sound too good to be true? While this example may seem a bit all-too-fantastic to some, it is my belief (and the belief of many other health experts) that using noni to complement a beneficial diet, regular exercise, stress reduction and an otherwise healthful lifestyle can produce such results.

Adding Up the Noni Numbers

To better learn how noni is being used today, and to learn of its efficacy in treating particular conditions, I conducted (and still am conducting) a statistical survey that offers a fairly accurate picture of noni's medicinal benefits. As of this writing, I have interviewed over 50 doctors and health professionals whose patients previously used or are now using noni to treat different conditions. What I've discovered is astounding: after reviewing the results of the more than 10,000 people using noni, I have determined that noni undoubtedly possesses a variety of efficacious medicinal properties that modern medicine cannot ignore.

What do the results reveal? While later chapters will discuss them in more detail, the following are some of the most impressive (keep in mind that nearly all the data comes from individuals using Tahitian Noni Juice™, a product marketed by Morinda, Inc.):

• Two-thirds (67 percent) of 847 people with cancer experienced significant lessening of their symptoms.
• Ninety-one percent who used noni juice noticed an increase in energy levels.
• Seventy-two percent of overweight patients lost weight.
• Eighty-seven percent of those drinking noni for high blood pressure experienced a significant drop in blood pressure.
• Nearly 90 percent of those with chronic pain experienced a significant decrease in pain.
• Eighty percent of arthritis sufferers reported a lessening of arthritic symptoms.
• Side effects among all participants were minimal or nonexistent.

While this survey was not a double-blind study, its results indicate that noni juice does possess some powerful and safe medicinal properties that merit further investigation. Furthermore, the writing of this book follows much in the same line. I have written a number of books, most dealing with mainstream health topics, for which I had at my disposal literally hundreds of studies, trials, published reports in scientific journals and the opinion of dozens of qualified and educated professionals. Compiling the information for these books was mostly gathering material, analyzing it, and organizing it into coherent, understandable text.

But this book is different. Because of the relative obscurity of noni, there are not, comparatively speaking, huge numbers of scientific reports on noni's health benefits, its safety, or how it is best used. In fact, most of the material that I have compiled in order to write this book is not found in prestigious scientific journals, nor is it the result of years-long scientific studies costing millions of dollars. Gathering material on noni and other natural therapies has been a bit like learning to ride a bike. Though the amount of research on natural remedies has been accelerating recently, much of it is published in foreign journals, some not translated into English, or simply not reported in mainstream medical databases. Nor are there the familiar foundations of medical expertise in academic settings to initiate, confirm and explore further the emerging theories about natural products like noni.

So, my investigations went beyond just the conventional medical realm. I reviewed anything I could get my hands on that might give me better insight into the therapeutic actions of noni. I interviewed doctors, their patients and others who were currently investigating noni as a medicinal agent. I have spoken with leading herbalists and others in "natural" health fields. I have reviewed popular publications and tracked every legitimate lead regarding the use of noni.

My experience at times has been somewhat discouraging and disheartening. All too many individuals excited about promoting noni to their friends, family and others, have made outrageous claims regarding noni, making it into a "miracle medicine" that can cure just about any ailment. Conversely, I encountered stiff resistance from acquaintances to the idea that a tropical fruit could provide valuable health benefits. Doctors and other health professionals whom I thought might have an open mind to a new and exciting nutritional supplement have simply dismissed it as an over-hyped fruit juice.

On the other hand, the experience has also been inspiring, enlightening and fulfilling. I have seen the dramatic recovery of a woman from the debilitating effects of chronic fatigue syndrome after incorporating Tahitian Noni Juice™ into her life. Compelling was the account I received from a Gulf War veteran, whose entire family was suffering from various conditions, yet experienced dramatic improvement after beginning a regimen of noni use. I was especially pleased to learn of an elderly couple's success in using noni juice to treat cataracts and arthritis. I've had conversations about, received correspondence regarding, and otherwise witnessed the magnificent changes in the lives of individuals who have not only used noni to reverse specific health conditions, but also made the necessary modifications in their general lifestyle to positively affect their health.

Noni: Rally Point in the Health Revolution

As mentioned earlier, one of the main focuses of this book will be that of how to effectively incorporate noni into a holistic health plan. That is, a plan that treats the whole body—the mind, the spirit, the emotional and the physical. Since medicine began narrowing its focus on developing drugs as the primary weapon against disease, interest in how the health of the entire body is affected has waned. Early traditional healers (in this case, I mean "traditional" to refer to those native or folk healers who were their societies' principal health care providers before the emergence of allopathic medicine) were very interested in the body as a whole. They viewed the body primarily as an organism whose various systems interacted in a complex and interwoven manner. What happened in the digestive system could very well affect the cardiovascular system; how a person felt emotionally on a particular day could determine whether he or she experienced heartburn that night.

The Return of the Holistic Healer

Over the last several decades, Western medicine has diverted from the basic philosophy of holistic healing. Doctors have been trained that each of the body's systems is largely self-contained. What happens in the digestive system generally doesn't have much to do with the rest of the organism. Pharmaceutical "medicines" are a focal point in the training and development of the industry. Typically, the primary function of many drugs today is only to mask the symptoms of a particular condition, not to eliminate its cause. As mentioned earlier, because of the innate need for us all to have good health, the research into and development of synthetic drugs and medical procedures has evolved into one of the most lucrative and powerful industries in North America and beyond. It's no secret to anyone that taking one, two, three, or even more pills a day for our various complaints is not only common, but also acceptable.

Nonetheless, a health revolution is under way. Recent years have seen significant changes in this philosophy. Doctors and health care professionals are beginning once again to return to the basic notion that the body is a complex organism that needs complete, or holistic, care to ultimately achieve greater health. And noni can play an integral part in such a holistic health-care plan.

HOW CAN NONI IMPROVE MY HOLISTIC HEALTH PLAN?

Our earlier scenario of how noni can help one become more healthy and ultimately enjoy a fuller life may seem to some to be a bit extreme. However, I firmly believe in the adage, "An ounce of prevention is worth a pound of cure." In this case, even taking noni in small doses (such as one ounce) can help relieve already existing symptoms as well as prevent the onset of others. I have been involved in literally hundreds and hundreds of cases where Tahitian Noni Juice™ brought about sometimes subtle, and sometimes dramatic changes in their health. About now, you may be asking yourself, "How exactly can noni help me?" The following examples illustrate just some of the ways in which noni can really improve one's quality of life.

Increased energy levels. For centuries, noni was used as a food staple in Polynesian and other cultures, and in times of famine because of its high nutrient content. Current research has verified that noni is, indeed, extremely nutritious. Moreover, modern-day use has shown that a large majority of those taking noni for a specific health condition (other than fatigue or lack of energy) also experience a notable increase in their energy levels. (Later sections of this book will highlight some of these individuals.)

Relief from chronic and severe pain. Pain, whether a symptom of a known malady or simply chronic in nature, is one of today's most debilitating health conditions. When I was a practicing medical doctor, one of the most common complaints issued to me by patients was that of chronic, bothersome and constant pain. Noni's ability to relieve pain, whether from chronic backaches or from arthritis in the joints, has long been recognized. In fact, *Morinda citrifolia* carries the self-explanatory title "pain-killer" in various cultures. Though the mechanisms that noni employs to reduce pain aren't completely understood, there is no doubt that noni can profoundly impact both the severity and chronic nature of various types of pain. (Later sections will discuss this more in depth.) Among the thousands of cases involving Tahitian Noni Juice™ that I have reviewed, relief from pain is one of the most commonly reported benefits.

Stimulation and strengthening of the immune system. This is one of the most intriguing areas concerning noni's amazing health benefits. As previously mentioned, noni was used historically by the various island cultures to treat numerous health conditions. Of course, these people did not understand how noni worked. However, present-day research has discovered that noni possesses the ability to stimulate and enhance the body's immune functions. For instance, a study conducted by researchers at the University of Hawaii discovered that noni effectively aids the body in fighting cancerous growths by activating the body's production of nitric oxide (NO), cytokines, and other agents that actively seek out and destroy cancerous cells. Other research indicates that noni possesses potent antimicrobial properties (for instance, it has been shown to fight the dreaded *E. coli* bacteria).

Increased levels of physical activity. While there is currently more awareness regarding the benefits of increased exercise and healthy

"I Can Play Tennis As Frequently As I Want!"

Carolyn Riley explains how noni helped her experience a remarkable recovery from several health conditions:

"As an adolescent, I began having knee trouble. My kneecaps would subluxate (slip out of alignment) and cause me excruciating pain. As a young adult, I had recurring knee problems which seemed to be worsening, twice having knee injuries requiring weeks of immobilization and subsequent physical therapy.

"Although I recovered from those injuries, my knees would sometimes 'catch' or even lock up. For 12 years, from age 40 to 52, I suffered from chronic swollen knees and resulting stiffness and pain.

"I am an avid tennis player, playing several times a week. My bad knees rarely kept me from playing, but they caused me much pain and made me feel older and more tired than a person my age should. Getting out of my car, or climbing or descending stairs, or rising from a movie seat, or running for a tennis ball, I was constantly reminded by the stiffness and pain of my bad knees.

"In 1985 I had X-rays and an MRI to see what was causing the problem. Surgery was not indicated, but as my doctor put it, I did not have 'the knees of a spring chicken.' He prescribed exercises to strengthen the muscles that help hold the kneecaps in place. This was to prevent further injury, but it did nothing to reduce the swelling and pain I was experiencing.

"In April of 1997, a former high school classmate told me about noni juice. I began to take one ounce a day. After three weeks, my knees stopped swelling and were pain-free. I have had no swelling, stiffness, or pain in my knees since May of 1997. I am more mobile on the tennis court, can play as frequently as I want and for longer periods of time. I feel as if I have a new pair of legs, and I certainly feel younger and better than I did for those 12 years when I actually was younger.

"I still only take one ounce a day because I have had such good results with that dosage although I know others who choose to take more. Over time, I have noticed additional benefits from using noni. My fingernails are stronger than before; I have less anxiety; both my reading and distance vision have improved. After taking noni for seven months, I was alerted by my hairstylist that I had new hair growth all over my scalp. In addition, I recently realized that the dark pigmentation along my jawline, which appeared years ago when I began hormone replacement therapy, has faded to normal again. I believe that Tahitian Noni Juice™ has improved my body's ability to absorb what it needs from the nutrition and supplements I take. My body has responded by restoring and repairing itself better than ever!

"Although other testimonies may be more dramatic than mine, I cannot overemphasize how noni has improved the quality of my life. I thank God for noni juice."

dietary habits, we often subject ourselves to more stress than ever before, and thus begins the vicious cycle: our energy begins to wane, so we don't exercise as much, which leads us to feel depressed, which often makes us eat more, resulting in weight gain, etc. Noni can kick our energy levels up a notch, giving us an impetus to get out and do something. Noni also helps relieve the debilitating effects of conditions that limit physical activity, such as arthritis, fibromyalgia, autoimmune disorders, and chronic fatigue syndrome. Noni could provide the launch pad for a cycle that leads us back once again to vibrant health.

Relief from and prevention of a wide array of health disorders. This point is clear: noni has been used for thousands of years (and is still being used) to treat an impressive variety of health conditions. Centuries of common use, coupled with modern scientific research, shows that noni is undoubtedly a powerful medicinal agent.

How is it possible that noni can work against so many diseases and health conditions? As we'll investigate further in the book, Dr. Ralph Heinicke has put forth the well-researched theory that noni contains the necessary ingredients for the body to make xeronine, a substance he and other scientists and health professionals believe allows the body's cells to maintain normal function. Without xeronine, cells will begin to falter in their various responsibilities. Ultimately, these "sick cells" (a term I coined some years back which describes cells that are not functioning properly) contribute to the onset of disease, be it high blood pressure, diabetes, arthritis, or cancer. Research also indicates that in the case of cancer, noni can kick-start several of the body's own defense systems to counteract cancerous growths. Another example involves hypertension, or high blood pressure. Research data published by researchers in Hawaii reveals that noni provides the body with nitric oxide, a valuable substance that allows blood vessel walls to relax and expand, lowering high blood pressure and helping with a variety of other cardiovascular problems. (Just as a side note, nitric oxide has recently attracted large amounts of attention because researchers investigating its health benefits won the Nobel prize for medicine in 1998.)

It's no secret that even the most simple of ailments, such as the common cold, can make life miserable. Because of noni's nutritional and therapeutic qualities, one can more effectively fight any condition that may arise and be well on the way to an improved state of health.

Chapter Summary Points

- When incorporated into a well-designed health plan, noni can work wonders in relieving symptoms of numerous disorders, preventing others, and promoting overall improved health.
- My survey of more than 50 doctors and health professionals and more than 10,000 noni users found that noni was able to positively affect a large majority of conditions. This survey has convinced me that noni undoubtedly possesses a variety of medicinal properties that modern medicine cannot ignore.
- In general terms, noni can enhance one's life by increasing energy levels, relieving chronic pain, strengthening the immune system, allowing for more physical activity, and preventing the onset of various health diseases and disorders.

How Is Noni
Used Today?

I HAVE COVERED briefly the history of noni—where it comes from, its use as a food and dyeing product, and most importantly, its spectacular track record as a healing agent. I've also discussed how the Western world is in the midst of a health revolution, moving from an almost exclusive reliance on conventional medicine to a more complete and holistic approach. With this revolution has come the emergence of noni as a safe and natural health supplement.

The Arrival of Noni to the U.S.

As the world becomes "smaller" and more interconnected, information and knowledge become more readily available. Consequently, it's safe to say that the existence of a legitimate health-promoting agent like noni could not remain a secret forever. And it hasn't.

In 1994, two prominent food scientists—John Wadsworth and Stephen Story—were introduced to the island fruit *Morinda citrifolia*. They were educated as to its uses, both as a coloring substance and as a medicinal agent, and to its rich history in various cultures throughout the world. Their interest piqued, they began to more fully investigate this plant, its fruit and its potential to be developed and marketed as a legitimate health supplement to the rest of the world.

They were soon able to appreciate how valuable noni is. They pursued their investigation into the harvesting and processing of a noni juice product that both was palatable (remember noni's somewhat foul taste) and that preserved its most important nutritious and medicinal properties.

Though Story and Wadsworth were relatively successful in developing a process that ensured a high-quality product, they were still lacking one thing—someone who could take their product and successfully market it to the United States as well as the rest of the world.

They soon had their answer. Kerry Asay, a former CEO of one of the world's most successful and oldest network marketing companies, determined that noni did indeed represent an exciting and promising medicinal agent. With the help and expertise of a few other individuals, Asay teamed up with his brother, Kim Asay, Wadsworth and Story to form Morinda, Inc., a company whose purpose was to help develop and distribute the first available commercial noni product. Shortly after, they convinced Kelly Olsen, an experienced marketer, to share their vision and join the team.

Needless to say, they have been very successful. In 1996, the first commercial noni product, developed and marketed by Morinda and called Tahitian Noni Juice™, was shipped to the United States. Since then, Morinda has been the undisputed leader in both the development and sale of noni products. But theirs is not the only success. As of this writing, there are a number of other companies that have developed noni products with the hope of capitalizing on its growing popularity.

In the meantime, other notable professionals in the scientific and medical world have involved themselves in research concerning noni's health benefits. Individuals like Ralph Heinicke, Ph.D., the initial and principal pioneer in noni research, and Anne Hirazumi, Ph.D., who has continued Dr. Heinicke's work, have also greatly contributed to the growing interest in noni as a legitimate and safe botanical healing agent.

It is no secret that the general noni market, both here in the U.S. and worldwide, has virtually exploded. Which brings us to the question of how, in light of its popularity, noni is being used in the U.S. and worldwide.

Abdominal pains	Abdominal swelling
Abscesses	Anticancer activity
Antibiotic and Antimicrobial	Arthritis
Backache	Balanced nutrition
Burns	Chest infections
Dark spots on skin	Deficient Macrophages
Depression	Diabetes (Type 2)
Diaphragmatic hernia	Diarrhea
Dry or cracked skin	Eye complaints
Heart disease	High blood pressure
Infection of mouth/gums	Inflamed, sore gums
Inhibits early chronic fatigue synd.	Intestinal worms
Regulates thymus	"Sick People Syndrome"
Sore throat with cough	Stroke
Tonic after childbirth	Toothaches
Tuberculosis	Urinary tract ailments
Virus problems	Wounds, fractures

Table 3.1: **Some scientifically documented conditions for which noni has been used.**

My Survey: Over 10,000 Points of Proof

Shortly after noni products arrived in the U.S. and Canada, I was asked by a publisher with whom I was working at the time if I knew anything about a medicinal plant/fruit called noni. Though I hadn't, I agreed to initiate research to see what I could find. Initially, I did not find many people who knew much about noni, though the few I did find and talk to were very passionate about its reputed health benefits. A few days after my agreement to investigate noni, I was conversing with some good friends of ours, Warren and Laurelle Turski. Shortly into our conversation, Laurelle began describing an amazing medicinal plant she had been using that supposedly possessed a fairly impressive therapeutic arsenal. "What was it?" I asked. "Noni," she replied.

If I hadn't been initially intrigued by this tropical fruit with the funny-sounding name, my interest now grew by leaps and bounds. I felt I was onto something that not many knew about, but which could

"Noni Couldn't Do Anything But Help"

Gayle Holdman explains how noni provided her with some much-desired benefits:

"In 1996 I was introduced to noni juice and its wonderful health benefits. At the time, I had no idea what it would do for me but I just felt there was something special about this particular product. Because it was so perfectly natural I felt it was something that I could add to my diet without any fear of side effects. It couldn't do anything but help.

"So I started taking noni faithfully every day. I would take one ounce in the morning and one ounce in the evening. And after two weeks, I began my menstrual period, which was very strange because normally I have strong symptoms of PMS leading up to my period. This time, I had none. My period had always been extremely irregular and the only time I knew when it was coming is when I would have a terrible day of PMS stress, emotional headaches, and a number of other horrible symptoms.

"The fact that noni helped eliminate my PMS made me very excited. Then, after I counted up the days between periods, I realized that it had been exactly 28 days. Like I said, that had never, ever happened to me.

"At that point I had been married almost four years. My husband and I had never been able to have children. Right after regulating my menstrual cycle, I became pregnant for the first time. I'm certain it was the noni juice that helped to put me on a correct cycle, which ultimately helped me get pregnant.

"So now we have our baby boy. He is extremely healthy, and we absolutely love him. He has been our greatest blessing, and we have noni juice to thank for that."

be extremely valuable not only to me and my family, but to the entire world. My investigation became more serious, more urgent. Soon enough, I had spoken with enough doctors, health professionals, medical patients, and other individuals who had used noni to treat their specific conditions, to see that noni was indeed a promising nutritional supplement. As the months passed, I determined to conduct a well-organized and specific survey as to how noni was being used, its success, and its safety and side effects.

Consequently, over the last three years I have collected data from over 50 doctors and more than 10,000 patients/individuals taking noni. This information has contributed to a formidable database of how noni is currently used.

THE SURVEY RESULTS

To answer the question, "How is noni used today?" I am providing a comprehensive overview of the results of my survey, which demonstrate quite decisively that noni can be used safely and successfully for a wide array of health problems.

Cancer. Despite significant advances in the treatment of cancer, it remains a menacing prospect for those who are faced with battling it. But there still is hope. Mounting evidence suggests that diet and lifestyle can play a huge part in both the prevention and treatment (whether sole or complementary) of various cancers. Amidst excitement over new treatments, noni has emerged as both a natural, safe and effective anticancer agent. Of all the significant research centered on noni, there is more investigation of its anticancer properties than any other area.

One of these principal studies, published in 1997, investigated the modes of action behind noni's apparent capability to fight cancer. Conducted by researchers at the University of Hawaii, the study found that in mice, noni can stimulate the immune system to increase its activity (specifically among many of the body's various defense cells). In the words of the researchers, after noni reached the cells, "the 'defense' cells were activated, many of the cancerous cells were killed, and tumor growth was significantly suppressed. This suggests that in mice, noni-ppt [noni precipitate] suppresses tumor growth by activating the host immune system rather than acting directly as a toxin." The researchers go on to conclude that "the administration of noni-ppt to mice with Lewis lung cancer resulted in a significantly enhanced survival rates . . . thus substantiating the theory that noni-ppt acts by stimulating the host immune system."[1]

In my survey, there were hundreds of individuals who took noni juice (in the form of Tahitian Noni Juice™) or are still taking it as part of their cancer-treatment regimen. More than two-thirds of over 900 cancer patients taking noni reported that it helped reverse or lessen their various symptoms of cancer. Susan of Houston, Texas, explains how noni helped her recover from her cancer:

> After my breast cancer resulted in me receiving a mastectomy, I soon discovered that the cancer had spread to my colon, spine and right kidney. I immediately underwent two weeks of chemotherapy, but because of the debilitating side effects, the doctor decided to discontinue that particular type of chemotherapy. He asked that I make an appointment to come back into his office for more testing and he would make the determination as to the type of chemotherapy I should get on. My appointment was made for ten days from then.
>
> In the meantime, a friend of mine contacted me and had just heard about noni juice. I was willing to try anything and figured I had nothing to lose at this point. I consumed substantial amounts of the juice, drinking several bottles during those ten days. The results were incredible. I felt so much better and had more strength and stamina than I remembered having in a long time. On the tenth day, I went back to the hospital for the required testing and then headed over to the doctor's office. The hospital had immediately sent the results to the doctor via the computer, so by the time I got there he was already aware of the outcome of the testing. When he came in to see me, he had the strangest look on his face. I felt I was doomed and he was going to tell me that I only had three weeks to live. What he said was that the testing showed no signs of cancer, and only a small spot on my right kidney, which was probably nothing more than a cyst at that point.
>
> We were both so taken by surprise, I still have problems believing it. I am still under the doctor's care, but I have gone back to working a 30-hour week and have my strength back. I now only take two ounces each day for maintenance. I don't ever want to be without this juice, because I truly believe I wouldn't be able to write this if I hadn't learned about the wonders of noni juice.

CONDITION	# WHO TOOK ONLY NONI	# HELPED
Cancer, lessened symptoms	9	5
Heart disease, decreased symptoms	13	8
Stroke	5	3
Diabetes, type 2	6	4
Energy, increased	18	14
Sex, enhanced enjoyment	5	4
Obesity, lost excess weight	24	15
Fuzzy thinking, helped clear	11	6
Smoking, stopped	24	13
Arthritis, lessened symptoms	42	29
Pain, including headaches, decreased	43	31
Depression, lessened symptoms	14	9
Allergy, decreased symptoms	8	5
Fibromyalgia, decreased symptoms	11	6
Digestion, improved	15	10
Breathing, improved	27	17
Cholesterol, lowered	16	14
Cluster headaches, reduced	19	10
Longer/stronger fingernails	5	3

Table 3.2: **Results of noni supplementation in persons who used no other food supplement or medication.** *It should be noted that 74 out of the 93 people who used only noni juice had two or more problems existing simultaneously that were helped by noni. Over half the people were clinically helped with one or more of their problems after taking nothing but noni.*

High blood pressure/vascular disorders. Because it is not clear why blood pressure rises to such abnormal levels as to be called "hypertension," it is conversely difficult to explain why noni may be able to help normalize blood pressure levels. There are, however, various well-respected and legitimate theories.

In 1992, Dr. Isabelle Abbott, a recognized expert in botanical sciences, noted that one of the more common uses of noni included controlling high blood pressure. Following Dr. Abbott's lead, I searched the literature to find which phytonutrients (foods with healing properties) in noni could possibly help lower high blood pressure to normal levels. I soon discovered that scopoletin, which is found in noni, dilates constricted blood vessels. When blood vessels are constricted and

CONDITIONS REPORTED TO RESPOND TO NONI	# WHO TOOK NONI FOR THAT CONDITION	% HELPED*
Cancer, lessened symptoms	847	67%
Heart disease, decreased symptoms	1,058	80%
Stroke	983	58%
Diabetes, Types 1 and 2	2,434	83%
Energy, increased	7,931	91%
Sexuality, enhanced enjoyment	1,545	88%
Muscle, increased body-building	709	71%
Obesity, lost excess weight	2,638	72%
High blood pressure, decreased	721	87%
Smoking, stopped	447	58%
Arthritis, lessened symptoms	673	80%
Pain, incl. headaches, decreased	3,785	87%
Depression, lessened symptoms	781	77%
Allergy, decreased symptoms	851	85%
Digestion, improved	1,509	89%
Breathing, improved	2,727	78%
Sleep, improved	1148	72%
Fuzzy thinking, helped clear	301	89%
Well-being, increased feeling of	3,716	79%
Mental acuity, increased alertness	2,538	73%
Kidney health, improved	2,127	66%
Stress, helped cope with	3,273	71%

Table 3.3: **Conditions helped by people who used noni juice (n=>10,000).** This table depicts the pooled percentage of people who experienced objective and/or subjective improvement of their symptoms after taking noni. The majority of noni users who did not get optimal results failed to do so because they took a smaller amount and/or took it for a shorter time than what was recommended, or simply did not respond for unknown reasons.

It should be noted that noni can be used together with all other medications because there are virtually no negative interactions. In some situations, noni can allow other medications to act more efficiently. You should tell your health professional that you are taking noni as your physician might want to decrease the dose of the medication prescribed. It should also be noted that side effects were minimal. Less than 5 percent had loose bowel movements, a slight belch or developed a mild rash. The belch and loose bowel movements disappeared when the dose was decreased. The rash cleared within 72 hours after the person stopped taking noni. Concerning use by pregnant or nursing women, noni has been reported to be safe.

more narrow, the heart has to work harder to distribute blood to the body. However, as a result of noni's relaxing of the vessels, a normalization of the blood pressure takes place, which ultimately leads to less wear and tear on the heart.

Even more exciting is the data showing that noni stimulates certain cells in the body to produce nitric oxide (NO), a substance that recently has attracted much attention due to its ability to relax blood vessel walls. So important has been the research into this substance that researchers investigating its use as a vasodilating agent won the Nobel prize for medicine in 1998. Again, since the causes of high blood pressure are still cloudy, it is difficult to absolutely assign an explanation as to how noni can help lower high blood pressure. Nevertheless, modern research—including studies conducted at Stanford University, the University of California at Los Angeles (UCLA), the University of Hawaii, Union College of London, and the University of Metz in France—indicates that noni may produce positive benefits when it comes to normalizing high blood pressure.

Noni has been shown to aid other disorders related to the heart and vascular system. For instance, my survey found that for the 983 patients who took noni to help recover from strokes, more than 55 percent reported that it helped in their recoveries. The survey also shows that about 80 percent of those individuals taking noni juice to relieve symptoms of heart disease reported that it did just that. And nearly three-fourths of those using noni to improve their mental acuity (which can definitely be affected by increased blood flow to the brain) indicated that using noni produced significant results for them.

Diabetes, Type II. Adult-onset diabetes is largely attributed to the decreasing ability of the body's cells to effectively utilize carbohydrates, protein, fats and energy. Conversely, noni reportedly possesses the remarkable ability to provide the body with the essential alkaloid xeronine, which helps repair dysfunctional cells that previously couldn't utilize energy effectively. I believe that xeronine is largely responsible for the the transformation of these "sick" cells to properly functioning cells that can adequately assimilate and utilize the body's available energy and thus relieve the symptoms of diabetes. The results of my survey are certainly convincing. Of the more than 2,500 patients with either Type I or Type II diabetes, almost 85 percent reported that they experienced a noticeable change in their condition after implementing a regimen involving noni juice.

Chronic pain. Most of us know that pain is a common companion to most maladies. Arthritis, headaches, cancer and neuromuscular disorders come packaged with the often severe side effect of pain. Sometimes it is subtle, other times it can be extremely debilitating. Noni, on the other hand, has been shown to readily combat pain associated with various disorders. In fact, there are many doctors familiar with noni who believe that pain relief is noni's most valuable health benefit, which corresponds with the notion that noni is commonly referred to as "pain-killer" in various cultures. However, in light of all of the positive feedback concerning noni's use as a pain-relief agent, there may arise the question as to whether noni is toxic and/or addictive. According to clinical studies, popular use, and my survey results, the answer to this question is a resounding "no."

In 1990, researchers investigating the use of noni as an analgesic (substance that reduces the body's ability to feel pain) found that "the administration of noni extract shows a significant, dose-related, central analgesic activity in mice." The same researchers also added that the noni did not exhibit any toxic effects. My survey of more than 10,000 noni users reveals that more than 85 percent of individuals taking noni (again, in the form of Tahitian Noni Juice™) for chronic pain, including headaches, experienced noticeable relief in their pain. Additionally, it has been my experience, as well as that of many other health professionals, that noni not only can relieve pain, but can often do it in a surprisingly fast manner.

John Wells, a religious counselor, details how noni helped him find relief from chronic pain. He explains:

> About twenty years ago, I was in an accident, and one of my vertebrae was badly smashed. Since then, my right arm is frequently numb and I have chronic shoulder pain on that side. In addition, I also have had considerable pain in my right hand, much like arthritis, and my feet

were very painful at night. About two months ago, I began taking noni juice, and I can remember only once or twice that my hand was even partially numb, and the aching in my shoulder is gone. An added benefit of taking noni is that I no longer have the fairly frequent headaches that I used to experience.

As I discussed earlier, pain is a common companion to a variety of ailments. My survey of more than 10,000 noni users shows that more than three-fourths of those taking noni to relieve their symptoms of arthritis did experience some degree of relief. Of course, one of the most common complaints associated with arthritis is pain. And cancer certainly is associated with high levels of pain. The survey reveals that noni juice was able to lessen the effects of cancer in approximately two-thirds of those taking it. And the list goes on. From ailments like bursitis to migraines to premenstrual syndrome, noni has been used successfully and safely to treat pain.

The results of my survey are indeed impressive. And they are supported by another study (albeit smaller) conducted by Mian-Ying Wang, M.D. In Dr. Wang's study, which consisted of 84 patients, more than 85 percent reported positive results from using noni for a total of 33 differing health conditions. And just like in my survey, reported side effects were extremely low. In fact, in this study, no side effects were reported.

After reviewing all of the feedback from the doctors, health professionals and individuals who have used noni for medical purposes, I conclude the following:

- Noni helps treat most ailments in a large majority (78 percent) of users.
- Noni usually exerts its effects quickly, with most people experiencing results within days to weeks. (However, you should commit to taking noni for six months before deciding how much it helps.)
- Noni is essentially nontoxic and side effects, if any, are minimal and completely reversible.
- Noni works synergistically with other food supplements and/or medications.

- Noni probably helps prevent the onset of various disorders.
- Noni is reported to be safe for virtually everyone, including children, pregnant and lactating mothers, and the elderly.

Chapter Summary Points

- After being introduced to noni in 1994, food chemists Stephen Story and John Wadsworth began developing a noni juice product with the hopes of marketing it successfully.
- Eventually, Story and Wadsworth teamed with Kim and Kerry Asay and Kelly Olsen to form Morinda, Inc., which would eventually create Tahitian Noni Juice™, today's most popular noni product worldwide.
- Shortly after being introduced to noni, I began investigating its therapeutic capabilities to see if the claims surrounding it were legitimate. This led to my collecting data from more than 10,000 noni juice users and more than 50 doctors and health professionals who were either using the juice or recommending it to others.
- The results of my survey are certainly impressive. More than 78 percent of all users reported some positive benefit from using noni. And the results varied widely—conditions from arthritis to cancer to chronic fatigue syndrome to diabetes have all been successfully treated with a noni juice regimen.
- A study headed by Mian-Ying Wang, M.D. substantiates the results of my survey. Her study showed that a large of percentage (86 percent) of patients taking noni for various health problems experienced positive benefits.

Noni's Key Components

REMEMBER OUR PREVIOUS discussion of why some medical truths, even though they have been proven beyond a doubt, take so long in becoming accepted by both the medical world and by the general public? One could say that this time frame applies to what I will term the "xeronine system," in which noni is intricately involved; to a substance called nitric oxide, finally coming into the public's eye after years of anonymity; and to scopoletin, a substance long suspected of wielding powerful health benefits but whose time in the spotlight has yet to come. Of course, these are not all of the compounds in noni that contribute to its overall health-improving capabilities. There are many others (as demonstrated by Table 4.1 in this chapter) that in some way probably contribute to noni's synergistic ability to improve one's health.

While the precise mechanisms and processes by which noni works are not entirely clear, noni does contain a number of substances— enzymes, vitamins, minerals, proteins, and among others a small amount of the alkaloid xeronine—that clearly play a pivotal role in maintaining good health. In addition, research suggests that different agents in noni may act in a synergistic manner to produce desirable effects. Of particular interest is how noni exerts its healing action as an adaptogen. That is, noni (or its specific components) is transported to the areas in the body where cells function abnormally and assists them in resuming normal function. Much of the research, particularly in the area of cancer, also indicates that it strengthens the immune system, regulating cell function and the regeneration of damaged cells. It is noni's apparent operation on the very basic and critical cellular level that makes it an extremely promising medicinal tool and a candidate to combat a wide variety of health conditions. To understand how noni works this way, we must focus our discussion on xeronine, nitric oxide, scopoletin and the many other compounds that provide noni with its powerful healing properties.

Dr. Ralph Heinicke and the Xeronine System

As stated earlier, noni has attracted much attention from nutritionists, doctors, and other health professionals because of some of its key components, namely proxeronine and xeronine. The story behind the discovery of xeronine, proxeronine and the so-called "xeronine system" can provide much of the foundation for the powerful medical claims surrounding noni.

FIRST THINGS FIRST: INVESTIGATING BROMELAIN

Despite noni's longtime popularity in Pacific cultures as a medicinal agent, until the last half of this century there was little available information, scientific or otherwise, on noni. In the early 1950s, while at the Pineapple Research Institute in Hawaii, Dr. Ralph Heinicke began to conduct research involving pineapple and its components. Soon after initiating the research, Dr. Heinicke isolated a substance that he called bromelain. His initial investigation of bromelain revealed little of significant worth; however, he began to receive reports from other researchers of specific unique and beneficial medicinal properties associated with bromelain extracts. So, he began to review his data in light of the new information he had received and eventually concluded that the bromelain extract must contain additional unknown ingredients that contributed to its specific actions. Consequently, Dr. Heinicke and his research team began more thoroughly investigating bromelain and the other possible ingredients in bromelain extracts that could be responsible for its potential health benefits.

After several years of meticulous and careful research, Dr. Heinicke was finally able to identify what it was that contributed to the bromelain extract's particular medicinal properties. What he discovered was a substance, called proxeronine, that when combined with other substances in the presence of the enzyme proxeroninase, formed the alkaloid xeronine. Needless to say, Dr. Heinicke was extremely excited at the discovery of this potentially valuable substance. However, what Dr. Heinicke didn't know was how proxeronine functions, and how it contributed to the bromelain extract's therapeutic actions. Years of working with the bromelain and later with the noni extracts have provided Dr. Heinicke and other researchers with a better picture of how proxeronine functions. Simply put, proxeronine is one of the key substances needed for the body to produce xeronine, the principal agent responsible for noni's impressive array of therapeutic abilities. Xeronine, through a series of biochemical processes, serves as an aid in helping abnormally functioning cells resume normal function, and assists normal cells in maintaining their normal behavior. It is its activity at the cellular level that allows noni to benefit the body in such a variety of ways.

An additional note of interest is that Dr. Heinicke also discovered that while Hawaiian pineapple plants do contain proxeronine, more importantly he found that noni is the richest known source of the substance. In fact, noni contains up to 40 times more proxeronine than ripe pineapple, its nearest "competitor."

POINTING THE WAY TO XERONINE

This brings us back to bromelain, the original reason that Dr. Heinicke began his investigation into noni. During Dr. Heinicke's initial stages of research, bromelain was found to help fight various diseases and ailments, including chronic pain, cancer, arthritis, and severe menstrual cramps. Moreover, bromelain's abilities to fight these conditions was attracting enough attention for several large pharmaceutical companies to seriously consider researching it. In fact, Dr. Heinicke reports that the director of one these pharmaceutical companies stated to him that the discovery of bromelain and its accompanying constituents ranked high on the list of major medical developments of the last 50 years.

As a result, Dr. Heinicke was invited to lead the double-blind study required by the FDA for the commercialization of bromelain. After

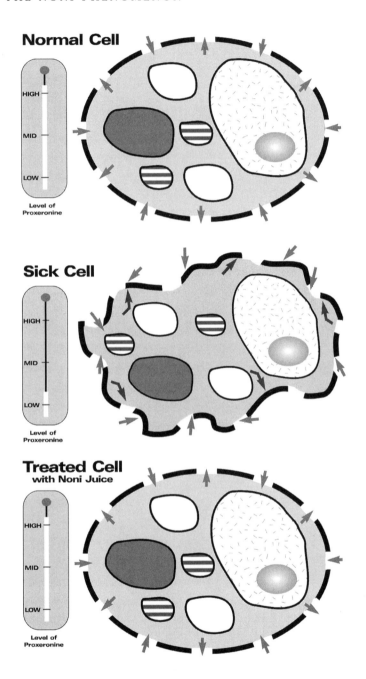

Figure 4.1: **How proxeronine from noni juice helps normalize the function of a "sick" cell.**

three months, the extensive tests revealed that purified bromelain and its protease enzyme (which the pharmaceutical company incorrectly believed to be the key component in this bromelain puzzle) had little or no pharmacological healing properties. Though not known to Dr. Heinicke and the company, the process used to isolate and purify bromelain had in fact removed the substance key to its active healing properties. Of course, we know now that substance was not protease, but proxeronine.

So, the natural course of action for the pharmaceutical company would be to determine why bromelain was ineffective after the purification process, right? Apparently not—for reasons concerning mainly financial risk, this company was dissuaded from further pursuing the research that could lead to a complete understanding of how and why bromelain worked as a therapeutic agent.

Thus, for the next 10 years, Dr. Heinicke continued his search for the secret behind bromelain and its mysterious constituents. He consulted with Gus Martin, the research director for a company that had meanwhile developed a bromelain tablet product. He and his company provided Dr. Heinicke (and others) with some groundwork data to further pursue the secrets behind bromelain. Dr. Heinicke also worked with Dr. Gerald Klein, who possessed extensive experience with burn patients in World War II, and who had devoted his time to finding more effective ways to treat burns. His work led him to bromelain and to Dr. Heinicke. Though they experienced some success, again they found that purified bromelain did little to aid the healing of burn patients. By this time, Dr. Heinicke was thoroughly convinced that purified bromelain was lacking a vital piece of the entire puzzle involving its dramatic pharmacological results.

The search by Dr. Heinicke and other researchers to determine why bromelain and its constituents worked paralleled the classic story of the five blind men who attempted to describe the nature of an elephant. Since each man felt only one part of the animal—a trunk, a foot, or a tail—consequently, they each had an incorrect perception of the entire animal. In this case, every specialized attempt to solve the puzzle resulted in an inaccurate picture of the whole.

Finally in 1974, Dr. Heinicke determined that the substance he had unknowingly isolated twenty years earlier and which he had regarded as simply an annoying contaminant was perhaps the key to understanding how bromelain could demonstrate pharmacological properties. As it turned out, this substance was proxeronine. Dr. Heinicke also concluded that another substance he had earlier isolated but disregarded in his research was indeed very necessary for the utilization of proxeronine. This substance was an enzyme that he called proxeroninase.

Over time, Dr. Heinicke clarified exactly what roles proxeronine, proxeroninase and a few other compounds play in producing beneficial medicinal effects. Dr. Heinicke ultimately found that these substances work synergistically to produce xeronine, which we know now to function adaptogenically in helping damaged and malfunctioning cells repair themselves and become healthy again.

Xeronine: A Cell's Best Friend

Knowing the basic history of proxeronine, we now turn our focus to xeronine, the final substance in this amazing process that contributes to the reversal of various health problems and the overall enhancement of one's health.

As stated earlier, the basic components involved in the body's biosynthesis of xeronine are proxeronine and proxeroninase (the enzyme required to catalyze the conversion process) and possibly various other compounds, such as vitamins, minerals, protein antioxidants and serotonin. Though the human body produces all of them, proxeronine is found in short supply.

So, how is xeronine produced in the body? According to Dr. Heinicke, the liver (which stores proxeronine) is signaled by the brain to release a "shot" of proxeronine into the bloodstream approximately every two hours. The various body organs and tissues can then take from the blood the proxeronine needed to produce xeronine for the repairing process. As I stated earlier, cells normally contain sufficient amounts of the other biochemical substance—proxeroninase—

required to synthesize xeronine; only proxeronine is limited in its supply. Ordinarily, the small amount of proxeronine the body harbors is enough to conduct the repairs needed by an average human. However, if there is a need for more xeronine in a particular organ—such as when precancerous cells are present, when there is a viral infection, or when there is an otherwise inordinately high level of stress—there usually is not enough proxeronine to accommodate this need. Consequently, one can see how noni, with its high levels of proxeronine, could be beneficial in filling this pressing need.

Realizing this, Dr. Heinicke endeavored to isolate pure xeronine from noni (xeronine is found in small amounts in noni). Achieving this result, he proceeded to use this purified xeronine in a series of trials involving mice given tetrodotoxin, an extremely potent toxin. Tetrodotoxin is commonly used in laboratory experiments to kill mice; its injection in mice results in a frenzied, spasmodic display that is immediately followed by death.

Dr. Heinicke administered to one group of mice pure tetrodotoxin, and to the other group both tetrodotoxin and xeronine. The results were dramatic, conclusive and even surprising to Dr. Heinicke. One hundred percent of those given only the poison died as expected—in the usual death throes and almost instantly. Conversely, 100 percent of those given both xeronine and the poison lived! And not only did they live, but they also displayed no outward signs of discomfort or trauma.

Dr. Heinicke repeated the trial several times to test its veracity. Each time, the results were the same. If ever there was a question in Dr. Heinicke's mind as to xeronine's pharmacological properties, there were none after this experiment.

Of course, proxeronine and xeronine are just two of the many health-promoting substances contained in noni or whose production is stimulated in the body by noni. However, as research by Dr. Heinicke and others suggests, they are two of the most important of noni's key components.

Nitric Oxide

As previously mentioned, another substance connected with noni's apparent health benefits is nitric oxide (NO), which may be best known to many as one of the ingredients in smog. In the body, however, nitric oxide is hardly a pollutant. Over the last several years, researchers have uncovered a series of revolutionary discoveries concerning NO and how critical it is to the function and action of a remarkable number of body systems. While noni does not contain nitric oxide, it has been shown in laboratory trials to stimulate the body to produce it. There have been literally thousands of research articles appearing in medical journals and text books since the biological role of nitric oxide was discovered in the 1980s—all of these paint a convincing picture that nearly everything the body needs to function correctly depends on the presence of NO. And now research has shown that noni, the "miracle" tropical plant, can stimulate the body to produce more NO, thereby preventing and helping control various disorders. Dr. Jonathan S. Stamler, a professor of medicine at Duke University, put it quite well when he said, "It [NO] does everything, everywhere. You cannot name a major cellular response or physiological effect in which it is not implicated today. It's involved in complex behavioral changes in the brain, airway relaxation, beating of the heart, dilation of blood vessels, regulation of intestinal movement, function of blood cells, the immune system, even how digits and arms move."[1]

Now, consider the various jobs that NO has been shown to perform inside the human body:

- It relaxes arteries, thereby contributing to normal blood pressure levels (which could otherwise skyrocket if it is in short supply).
- In promoting relaxed artery walls, it also keeps an adequate supply of blood coming to the heart, preventing angina pain (which results from an insufficient supply of oxygenated blood to the heart).
- It is a potent free radical scavenger that can contribute to lower cholesterol levels and prevents LDL cholesterol (the "bad" cholesterol) from oxidizing and becoming an even more dangerous substance.

- It inhibits premature coagulation in the blood, thereby preventing platelets from clumping together into clots that can cause heart attack and stroke.
- It enhances blood flow to the penis, helping to boost erections and to contribute to a more enjoyable sex life.
- It acts as a sort of ammunition for different immune system cells that use it to kill foreign bacteria, viruses and cancerous cells. (It has even been shown to shrink and destroy some types of tumors.)
- It is used by the brain to encode long-term memory and enhance blood flow to the brain.
- It functions as a "messenger molecule" that allows nerve cells in the body and the brain to communicate effectively.
- In addition to controlling "normal" hypertension, it can also serve to control high blood pressure brought on by pregnancy, a threatening condition to both mother and child.
- It aids in the regulation of insulin secretion by the pancreas, helping prevent and/or control diabetes.
- It provides the body with adequate stimulation to release the extremely important human growth hormone, a key to longevity as well as improvement in body composition by boosting lean muscle mass and bone density.

NITRIC OXIDE AND CARDIOVASCULAR HEALTH

As the above points illustrate, nitric oxide is heavily involved in many of the body's functions, but most importantly in cardiovascular function as well as immune function. However, it has only been recently that the arena of health professionals has come to accept this. The previous incredulity was understandable. Nitric oxide has escaped many physiologists' attention until now because it survives in the body for a mere five seconds or so, and because it bears no resemblance to any known biological regulator.[2]

However, a virtual tidal wave of information regarding NO has come forth, sweeping the worlds of modern medicine in just a few short years and making NO a new potential for improving health in broad-spectrum physiological terms. In 1992, nitric oxide was voted

"Molecule of the Year" by *Science* magazine, and consumer health publications began running articles with titles like, "Much Ado about NO" and "Say NO to Impotence!"

How, you may be asking, does nitric oxide help fight hypertension and other cardiovascular conditions? While later chapters of this book will describe this in more detail, I will now discuss in simple terms how the heart manages to effectively distribute blood to the entire body. Most of us know that at the center of the cardiovascular system is the heart, which branches off into the aorta, which then distributes the blood to the major arteries, then to smaller arterioles and finally to the tiny capillaries. The body regulates how these vessels contract and expand to either allow more blood flow or restrict it, depending on the body's needs. For instance, when one is jogging, several areas of the body, particularly the major muscles in the legs, need an increased oxygen flow to produce the needed contractions. On the other hand, if you are outside for extended periods on a cold winter morning, the core organs need increased blood flow to maintain the body's normal temperature.

All of this is achieved via two actions: vasodilation (opening up of the blood vessel—typically the arterioles—so more blood can flow through it) and vasoconstriction (closing of the vessel to decrease blood flow). And it is the smooth muscle rings around the blood vessel that perform these two actions. Imagine the blood vessel as a flexible garden hose that is surrounded by an ace bandage. Tighten the bandage and less water, or blood, is allowed to flow. Loosen the bandage and more can flow freely.

A variety of chemical signals can tell your smooth muscle "bandage" to relax or contract. Alcohol, for example, can temporarily relax smooth muscle, allowing blood vessels throughout the body to open up. This is one reason a shot of whiskey on a cold day can make your hands and feet feel warm (though it also increases the risk of hypothermia by not maintaining the temperature of your body's core organs).

On the other hand, when operating properly, the smooth muscle action in your vascular system is anything but arbitrary. It is, instead, a miraculous orchestration with nitric oxide being a principal instrument. This means that nitric oxide created by endothelial cells lining your vessels (which are stimulated by noni supplementation) is now known to be a major blood pressure regulator of the body's cardiovascular system.

So, although it is not known exactly how noni lowers blood pressure, improves recovery from stroke, or relieves symptoms of heart disease, it is clear from hundreds of years of common use, the thousands of users in my survey, and the mounting research into noni that its various constituents, like nitric oxide, can play an extremely active role in reversing diseases of the heart and vascular system and in promoting excellent cardiovascular health.

NITRIC OXIDE AND CANCEROUS CELLS

The body's various defense systems, often lumped together and given the umbrella term of "immune system," are a multifaceted and complex bunch of processes and agents. Most appreciated in these defense forces are the body's specialized "soldier" cells, such as natural killer (NK) cells that hunt down and destroy enemy invaders such as bacteria, viruses and cancerous cells. We also have a variety of phagocytes, which literally means "cell-eaters," including macrophages that gobble up, dissolve and spit out the few remains of attacking pathogens. There are also what may be referred to as "intelligence" cells that make note of the protein "uniforms" worn by invading cells so that next time they come around, the body's defense systems have designed a neutralizing antibody to render them ineffective.

In the mid 1980s, researchers were able to determine that macrophages—one type of the immune system's "cell-eaters"—had their own form of the enzyme that enables them to manufacture nitric oxide. In the coming years, more and more evidence surfaced that nitric oxide may well serve as a sort of "ammunition" that is capable of killing off microbial invaders and cancer cells alike. One good example of this was the published reports of a 1991 study in *The Lancet*, which showed that 30 grams of oral arginine (which the body uses to produce the NO) given to cancer patients over three days stimulated a 91 percent increase in the ability of their natural killer cells to neutralize cancerous cells.[3]

Noni and Nitric Oxide: Hand-in-Hand Partners

What is exciting and promising concerning the use of noni for strengthening the immune system is that recent scientific data has come to light that unmistakably shows that noni stimulates the body's biosynthesis of nitric oxide. A 1997 study from researchers at the University of Hawaii revealed that noni supplementation resulted in a substantial increase in macrophage activity (more than three times the normal). Additionally, when combined with interferon, another of the body's immune function substances, the effect was considerably increased. The researchers go on to recognize that "a series of cytokine assays and NO [nitric oxide] determination demonstrated that noni could stimulate the activation of macrophages. Noni effectively enhanced the production of NO. . ."[4] The notion that nitric oxide, whose biosynthesis is enhanced within the body, can be toxic to cancerous cells is extremely exciting.

Noni's activation of nitric oxide may not be confined to just battling cancer. There are numerous reports that indicate noni is a potent antimicrobial agent, effectively able to destroy various viruses and bacteria. Most intriguing is the notion that nitric oxide can again act as a deadly form of ammunition against invading pathogens. In some cases, nitric oxide gas interferes with iron-containing molecules crucial to cellular respiration. This kills the invader by poisoning its internal metabolism. Among the common infections that nitric oxide is known to treat by this mechanism are: Salmonella, the bacteria that results in numberless cases of food poisoning each year; E. coli, the infamous bacteria most often seen in food and other contamination cases; H. pylori, the same bacteria discovered by the Australian doctors trying to prove that ulcers were most often the result of bacterial infection; chlamydia, a widespread, sexually transmitted microorganism that results in anything from urethritis to sterility; and last, an overabundance of Candida albicans, which is the most common cause of yeast infection.

The second way nitric oxide neutralizes invading agents is by interfering with the enzymes necessary for DNA replication. By essentially throwing a "monkey wrench" into the actions of these necessary enzymes, nitric oxide can keep infectious agents (as well as many types of cancerous cells) from reproducing, which obviously limits their ability to injure the human body. There are numerous studies indicating that nitric oxide can indeed spur macrophages to disable cancer cells and invading pathogens. One study involving the use of a known carcinogen, showed that only 28 percent of rats given arginine (which the body uses to synthesize nitric oxide) developed cancer, while nearly 90 percent of rats not given arginine developed cancer. In addition, the cancerous growths in the arginine group were most commonly benign growths, while the growths in the control group were of a highly malignant form of cancer. Other studies have repeated nitric oxide's ability to completely destroy various bacteria, viruses and other dangerous microbes.

As early as 1963 was noni's ability to fight infectious organisms known. Oscar Levand, a researcher from the University of Hawaii, identified several dangerous pathogens against which noni was shown to be effective in neutralizing. His carefully constructed thesis states that "the medicinal value of the noni fruit was scientifically confirmed in vitro (in the test tube) by Bushnell and co-workers, who tested 101 Hawaiian plants for antibacterial activity. The juice of the noni fruit was found to be active against three strains of bacteria: *Staphylococcus aureus, Escherichia coli* and *Pseudomonas aeruginosa*. Antibacterial activity was also observed against five different strains of enteric pathogens: *Salmonella typhosa, Salmonella montevideo, Salmonella schottmuelleri, Shigella paradysenteriae BH* and *Shigella paradysenteriae III-z.*"[5] What must also be remembered is that noni can be doubly toxic to invading pathogens. Studies show that it can directly affect various bacteria; other additional research suggests that noni stimulates various processes in the body's defense system to further inhibit pathogenic activity.

As has been mentioned (and will be discussed further), research has clearly shown noni to be a stimulant in the production of nitric oxide in the body. In addition, other research has shown noni to be effective in killing various bacteria and viruses, including the deadly *E. coli*. Nitric oxide is just one of the many substances either contained in noni or whose synthesis is enhanced by noni that helps the body maintain basic functions and defend itself from unwanted and dangerous invaders.

(ethylthomethyl) benzene
1-butanol
1-hexanol
1-methoxy-2-formyl-3-hydrox-
yanthraquinone
2,5-undecadien-1-ol
2-heptanone
2-methyl-2-butenyl decanoate
2-methyl-2-butenyl hexanoate
2-methyl-3,5,6-trihydroxyan-
thraquinone-6-ß-primevero-
side
2-methyl-3,5,6-trihydroxyan-
thraquinones
2-methylbutanoic acid
2-methylpropanoic acid
24-methylcycloartanol
24-methylenecholesterol
24-methylenecycloartanyl
linoleate
3-hydroxyl-2-butanone
3-hydroxymorindone
3-hydroxymorindone-6-ß-
primeveroside
3-methyl-2-buten-1-ol
3-methyl-3-buten-1-ol
3-methylthiopropanoic acid
5,6-dihydroxylucidin
5,6-dihydroxylucidin-3- ß-
primeveroside
5,7-acacetin7-O-ß-D-(+)-glu-
copyranoside
5,7-dimethylapigenin-4'-O-ß-
D-D(+)=galactopyranoside
6,8-dimethoxy-3-methyl
anthraquinone-1,-O-ß-rham-
nosyl glucopyranoside
6-dodeceno-y-lactone
7-hydroxy-8-methoxy-2-
methylanthraquinone

8,11,14-eicosatrienoic acid
acetic acid
alizarin
alkaloids
anthragallol 1,2-dimethyl ether
anthraquinones
antrhagallol 2,3-dimethyl ehter
asperuloside
benzoic acid
benzyl alcohol
butanoic acid
calcium
campesteryl glycoside
campesteryl linoleyl glycoside
campesteryl palmitate
campesteryl palmityl glycoside
campestrol
carbonate
carotene
cycloartenol
cycloartenol linoleate
cycloartenol palmitate
damnacanthal
decanoic acid
elaidic acid
ethyl decanoate
ethyl hexanoate
ethyl octanoate
ethyl palmitate
eugenol
ferric iron
gampesteryl linoleate
glucose
glycosides
heptanoic acid
hexadecane
hexanamide
hexanedioic acid
hexanoic acid
hexose

Table 4.1: **Nutraceuticals identified in noni.**

hexyl hexanoate
iron
isobutyric acid
isocaproic acid
isofucosterol
isofucosteryl linoleate
isolaveric acide
lauric acid
limonene
linoleic acid
lucidin
lucidin-3- ß-primeveroside
magnesium
methyl 3-methylthio-
  propanoate
methyl decanoate
methyl elaidate
methyl hexanoate
methyl octanoate
methyl oleate
methyl palmitate
morenone-1
morenone-2
morindadiol
morindanigrine
morindin
morindone
morindone-6-ß-primeveroside
mucilaginous matter
myristic acid
n-butyric acid
n-valeric acid
nonanoic acid
nordamnacanthal
octadecenoic acid
octanoic acid
oleic acid
palmitic acid
paraffin
pectins

pentose
phenolic body
phosphate
physcion
physcion-8-O[{L-arabinopyra-
  nosyl} (1-3) {ß-D- g-D-
  galactopyranosyl (1-6) {ß-D-
  galactopyranoside}]
potassium
protein
resins
rhamnose
ricinoleic acid
rubiadin
rubiadin-1-methyl ether
scopoletin
sitosterol
sitosteryl glycoside
sitosteryl linoleate
sitosteryl linoleyl glycoside
sitosteryl palmitate
sitosteryl palmityl glycoside
sodium
sorandjidiol
ß-sitosterol
stearic acid
sterols
stigmasterol
stigmasteryl glycoside
stigmasteryl linoleate
stigmasteryl linoleyl glycoside
stigmasteryl palmitate
stigmasteryl palmityl glycoside
terpenoids
trioxymethylanthraquinone
undecanoic acid
ursolic acid
vitamin C
vomifoliol
wax

Table 4.1 (cont.): **Nutraceuticals identified in noni.**

Scopoletin: Noni's Other Blood Pressure Friend

Another of noni's apparent health-promoting agents, scopoletin was first isolated from noni in 1993 by researchers at the University of Hawaii. Following its initial discovery, additional researchers have suggested that scopoletin probably plays a key part in noni's ability to modify blood pressure. In 1992, Dr. Isabelle Abbott, a recognized expert in botanical sciences, noted that scopoletin was almost certainly involved in the body's response to noni's effect on hypertension.

As has already been mentioned, scopoletin could act synergistically to contribute to noni's adaptogenic effect: if the blood pressure is too high, it helps lower it; and if it is too low, scopoletin can help raise it. What is interesting is that animal studies have shown that scopoletin, when tested alone, may lower blood pressure to an unhealthy, or hypotensive, level. On the other hand, when tested in a noni extract, scopoletin appears to interact with other agents present in the extract to lower high blood pressure without bringing it too low. All in all, considering the available research, the results of my 10,000-patient survey, and the thousands of testimonials regarding noni use, I have not come across any documented evidence that noni can bring normal or high blood pressure to hypotensive levels.

Damnacanthal

Another constituent of noni believed to be responsible for at least some of the botanical's promising therapeutic effects is damnacanthal. Because it is generally accepted that noni does have a potent effect on the growth of cancerous tumors and cells, it can be assumed that damnacanthal plays a role in this process. In 1993, Hiramatsu and fellow researchers isolated damnacanthal from a chloroform extract of the noni root (remember that while the majority of noni products contain only juice from the noni fruit, there are a growing number of products that contain extracts from other parts of the plant in addition to the juice). These researchers' study revealed that damnacanthal was able to effectively inhibit cancer activity via regulatory signals in several human cancers, including lung, colon, pancreas and various leukemias. In other words, the researchers indicated that damnacanthal probably encourages cancerous cells to "believe" that they are in fact healthy cells, thereby stopping or at least slowing the otherwise accelerated multiplication of cells.[6]

The list could go on and on. As table 1 in this chapter indicates, there are literally hundreds of identifiable components of noni, many of which contribute to its spectacular ability to positively affect the human body. From nutrients like calcium and potassium to potent antibacterial agents like nitric oxide, noni possesses a wealth of valuable components that indeed make it a tropical wonder healer.

The Golgi Apparatus and the Heinicke-Solomon Theory

After reading about the "xeronine system" and the other compounds which noni either contains or of which it helps the body stimulate production, one may wonder as to the exact process used to utilize these compounds for health reasons. After reviewing the magnificent data of Dr. Heinicke and others, both he and I agreed on a working hypothesis that could adequately explain just how noni can be so effective in treating such a variety of ailments.

From his initial investigations into pineapple and bromelain to discovering the xeronine system and noni's apparent value as a medicinal agent, Dr. Heinicke has emerged as one of the principal pioneers in noni research. Earlier portions of this chapter reflect much of what Dr. Heinicke has discovered, revealing noni to have a wonderful array of disease fighting and health promoting benefits.

In spite of the work of Dr. Heinicke and others, there is still much that we don't understand about noni and its mechanisms of action. However, we have developed a "hypothesis" we have termed the "Heinicke-Solomon Theory."

So what does this theory entail? First, it has to do with something

1 *Noni juice, after being ingested, is broken down in the body.*

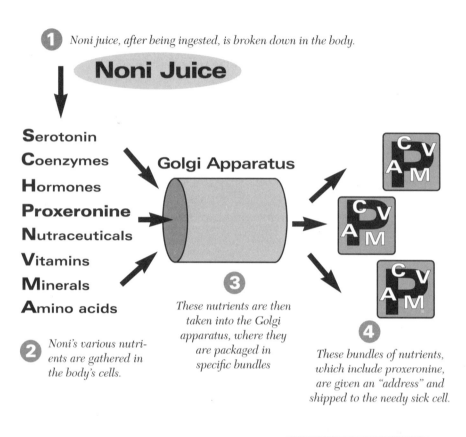

Noni Juice

Serotonin
Coenzymes
Hormones
Proxeronine
Nutraceuticals
Vitamins
Minerals
Amino acids

Golgi Apparatus

2 *Noni's various nutrients are gathered in the body's cells.*

3 *These nutrients are then taken into the Golgi apparatus, where they are packaged in specific bundles*

4 *These bundles of nutrients, which include proxeronine, are given an "address" and shipped to the needy sick cell.*

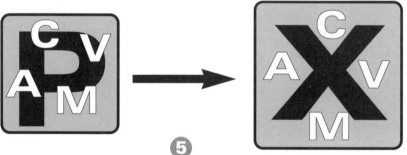

5 *When the proxeronine bundles are received by the damaged sick cell, it is then joined with enzymes and other nutrients to form xeronine, which is what the damaged cell ultimately uses to repair itself and regain normal function.*

Figure 4.2: **How proxeronine is converted to xeronine, which is then utilized by the body.**

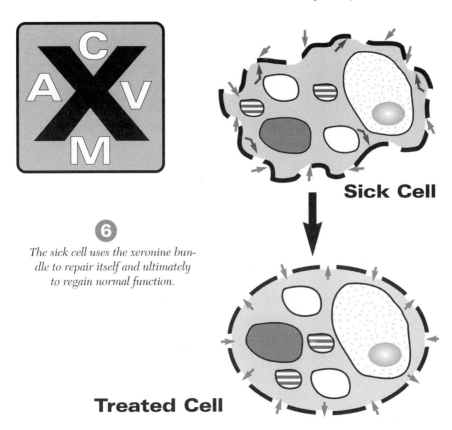

Sick Cell

⑥
The sick cell uses the xeronine bundle to repair itself and ultimately to regain normal function.

Treated Cell

Figure 4.2 (cont.): **How proxeronine is converted to xeronine.**

called the Golgi apparatus (GA). Known to exist since the late 1880s, the Golgi apparatus is found in most of the body's cells, and comprises an irregular network of layered tubes near the nucleus of each cell. Since their discovery, the exact function of the Golgi apparatus has been better understood, though there is still much that modern science does not know concerning it.

Simply stated, the principal function of the Golgi apparatus is as an assembler to package and ship various compounds, such as proteins, to other cells that need them. It is a fascinating process that resembles a very effective post office of sorts—each package is "labeled" and "delivered" to the intended cell address, after which the contents of the package are incorporated into the cell and utilized as needed.

Let's bring noni into this theory. When noni is consumed, its various components are incorporated into the body. One of these, proxeronine, travels to the cytoplasm of a specific cell and accumulates in the Golgi apparatus. Within the GA, proxeronine combines with the other biochemicals and building blocks the body uses to help maintain efficient and properly functioning cells. These biochemicals would include hormones, proteins, enzymes, serotonin, vitamins, minerals, antioxidants, and various others. The combination of proxeronine with these other compounds are specific and varied, according to the need of the cell to which they are being sent. The Golgi apparatus then assembles the necessary ingredients into a "package," gives it an "address" for its own cell or for another cell and delivers it via the bloodstream to the "sick" cell. As the package is opened, the proxeronine combines with a specific enzyme, proxeroninase, and is converted to xeronine. Xeronine then works with the other necessary biochemicals to create the required adaptogenic compound for that particular cell, allowing the cell to repair and regenerate itself. It is within this process that the cells regain their state of homeostasis (balance), which ultimately leads the body to an overall balanced state.

Of course, the limiting factor in this process is the proxeronine, which fortunately can be replenished by consuming adequate amounts of noni. The more "sick" or damaged a cell, the greater the amount of noni will be required to repair that cell. It is also very obvious that different cells from different organs and tissues will have specific and varying needs to both maintain normal function and to undertake any repairs it may need.

Elsewhere in the book, I discuss the relationship between *Morinda citrifolia* and nitric oxide. I mention that the 1998 Nobel prize for medicine was awarded to three doctors for their work on nitric oxide, and that their research would better help our understanding of how noni helps the body heal itself.

Of course, the preceding section explains how proxeronine from noni could combine with the necessary nutraceuticals, including protein, to be shipped to "sick cells." This bundle of nutrients is packaged by the Golgi apparatus, which puts the cellular address on it and ships it with specific protein within the cell itself or through the blood to specific "sick cells" elsewhere to help them repair themselves. Just prior to this writing, the 1999 Nobel prize in medicine was awarded to Rockefeller University biologist, Dr. Guenther Blobel. Dr. Blobel discovered the "postal system" that allows protein to be sent to cells using a "zip code," similar to what we postulate concerning proxeronine combining with various nutrients, including protein, to be sent and delivered to a damaged cell.

As we discuss in numerous sections of this book, noni appears to have a wide ranging ability to help relieve symptoms of various ailments, from chronic pain to diabetes to hypertension. It may be difficult for a sensible individual to believe that a plant or fruit could really be effective against so many health conditions and work for so many people. However, it is the understanding of how the Golgi apparatus works that makes this notion not only possible, but very exciting as well.

Chapter Summary Points

- While the precise mechanisms and processes by which noni works are not entirely clear, noni does contain a number of substances—enzymes, vitamins, minerals, proteins, and among others a small amount of the alkaloid xeronine—that clearly play a pivotal role in maintaining good health.
- Dr. Ralph Heinicke, the pioneering researcher into noni's health-promoting benefits, discovered the "xeronine system," which involves the combination of proxeronine, proxeroninase and other possible biochemicals to form xeronine, which is needed by the body's cells to help maintain their normal function. Noni contains all of these substances and can help the body increase its supplies of xeronine.
- Noni also helps stimulate the production of nitric oxide (NO), a valuable substance that provides the body with numerous benefits. Nitric oxide can strengthen the immune system by stimulating the production of and the action of various of the body's immune cells. It also has been shown to be instrumental in the lowering of high blood pressure and the improvement of overall cardiovascular health.

• Noni contains other substances, such as scopoletin and damnacan-thal, which provide other valuable benefits for improved health.

• Noni's success in alleviating various health conditions may be inter-twined with the function of the Golgi apparatus. The Golgi appara-tus functions primarily as an assembler to package and ship various compounds, such as proteins, to cells that need them. It is a fasci-nating process that resembles a very effective post office of sorts—each package is "labeled" and "delivered" to the intended cell address, after which the contents of the package are incorporated into the cell and utilized as needed.

• The "Heinicke–Solomon Theory" (developed by Dr. Heinicke and myself) postulates that the xeronine system may work hand in hand with the Golgi apparatus in helping "sick" cells to become well again. This could explain why noni is reportedly effective against such a wide variety of ailments.

Noni and Cancer

TERRY'S LIFE WAS like many others—mother of three, insurance claims representative, weekends cleaning and going to her kids' soccer games. Unknown to her, she matched the profile for breast cancer. At age 45, Terry was informed that the lump in her breast was cancerous—words she never imagined would be directed to her.

If you're like Terry, you probably have lived the majority of your life thinking that your chances of developing cancer were "one in a million." The fact is, every year more than one million Americans find they have cancer. This equates to a chance of about one in three that you will one day either die of cancer or become a cancer survivor.

Cancer is scary. It is often thought of as one of the most menacing and deadly of diseases. While it can be deadly, more research and knowledge, coupled with the individual's efforts to become educated, have given new hope to cancer patients. Though the number of cancer cases has not dropped, the success rate for overcoming cancer has seen a slow rise over the years. Simply stated then, there is a better chance now than ever before that Terry will overcome her cancer.

There are a number of reasons for the increasing success of doctors and scientists in fighting cancer: new drugs, better and earlier detection methods, more effective diagnostic methods, and a better understanding of how the body can naturally fight cancer.

However, before we examine noni's potent anticancer properties, it would be helpful to review some background material concerning cancer and its relation to you and me.

Are We in the Middle of a Cancer Epidemic?

With all the exposure cancer receives from the media, one might think that we were in the midst of an epidemic. While there are some worrisome statistics, it is evident that we aren't quite yet there. Mortality rates from cancers across the board actually have risen slightly during the forty-year period from 1950–1990, though most of that rise can be attributed solely to lung cancer. If lung cancer is not included in the equation, then mortality from cancer is actually down approximately 15 percent during that time, according to figures from the American Cancer Society.

Given the amount of research and funding, coupled with the "advancements" in cancer detection and treatment, you might think that deaths from cancer should have declined steadily. However, this hasn't happened. There are many reasons for this, probably many more than we can adequately discuss here. The most prominent of these, though, is that we live longer, thereby giving more time for diseases such as cancer to develop.

We all have to die of something. We've been remarkably successful at reducing the incidence of various diseases, so given that we all have to pass on somehow, as one mortality rate falls, another will automatically rise. This does not mean that you automatically will get cancer as you age. Cardiovascular disease is still the number one killer of Americans. There are innumerable health experts who believe that through simple changes in diet, nutrition and lifestyle we may extend our life expectancy by many years, effectively warding off diseases such as cancer that may well have come our way had we not decided, say fifteen years ago, to cut out red meat and begin exercising regularly. It is in this context—as part of a holistic health plan that focuses on all parts of health—that I want to discuss noni and its ability to fight cancer.

Noni and Cancer: Waging the Cell War

Carcinogenesis, the term describing the cancer process, translates from the Latin as "birth of the crab," and describes what these ancient people saw as a crab clawing its way through the body, taking over organ after organ, and devouring the victim piecemeal. The ancients had no idea why it happened, and were helpless to really do anything about it. Today we know the basics of why and how it happens (though all the details aren't so clear), and we certainly aren't helpless to do anything about it.

Cancer is a disease of the cells—all of the more than one hundred known cancers begin with one cell that mutates and eventually leads to wild cell proliferation. That single cell somehow evades the body's defenses and replicates unchecked. These newly formed cells can ultimately travel throughout the body, commandeering organs, diverting energy supplies, and eventually killing the "host"—us.

Are you aware that right now, as you read, your body is fighting off cancer on literally thousands of fronts? Each of our cells is bombarded daily with thousands of carcinogenic compounds, many of which are by-products of life itself. In fact, some experts put the number of "hits" by carcinogens against our body at literally trillions daily.

The point here is that cancer is principally a disease of the cell. Conversely, one of noni's strongest health benefits is its ability to work at the cellular level, helping abnormally functioning cells (like cancerous cells) to once again regain normal function and to stimulate the body's immune system to fight invading pathogens. Thus sparks the excitement of a growing number of health experts over noni's apparent ability to both prevent and reverse cancer.

The Immune System and Cancer

Some of the most exciting news from the world of cancer research revolves around immunotherapy, or encouraging the body's immune system to battle the disease. Most people have a basic knowledge of

A Short History of Cancer

Cancer is by no means a modern illness, though many refer to it as the disease of industrialization and urbanization. Evidence of cancer has been found dating back to the dawn of time, in fossils of animals and in mummified human remains.

The first historical reference to cancer dates back to the legendary Greek physician Hippocrates, around 400 B.C. While Hippocrates and his colleagues knew nothing about cells, they did understand that some growths were benign, or self-limiting, and that others were malignant, clawing their way through the body and consuming everything in their path until the host, or victim, died.

Cells were first seen by human eyes in 1665 when scientist Robert Hook examined a piece of cork under an early model of the microscope. He named the individual chambers he saw in the cork cells because they reminded him of the separate cells of a jail. Aided by microscopes, physicians later began to understand that cancer was a disease of the cells. In the nineteenth century, German physiologist Johannes Müller noted that the cells in cancerous tumors appeared to be quite different from normal cells. He found that they were as "hungry" and as rapidly growing as those found in developing embryos.

Much of the history of cancer occurrence among early civilizations is simply speculation. Some maintain that cancer was rare among the hunter-gatherer and pastoral peoples living in remote areas of the world when first visited by European explorers. From this has emerged the notion that cancer is primarily a modern disease, sprung out of industrialized civilization.

But there is another possible explanation: If indeed our hunter-gatherer ancestors were rarely faced with the prospect of cancer, it was probably due more in part to their diet and high levels of physical activity than to industrialization. Their diet would consist of high levels of fresh vegetables, fruits, roots, nuts, seeds, whole grains, almost no simple sugars, and lean meat. Because hunting and gathering requires a lot of time, energy and exertion, obesity would be almost nonexistent—it's hard to gain weight when you have to chase breakfast, lunch *and* dinner.

the immune system—essentially, that it is the principal tool in the body's fight against disease. The ways in which the immune system functions, however, can be extremely complex. We've all heard of T-cells, natural killer cells, interferon, macrophages, etc. These are all key players on the immune system's team, yet they comprise only a fairly small part of it.

So how does noni enhance the function of and strengthen the immune system? There are several theories—all of them exciting and promising—but one is attracting particularly strong attention. This theory centers on noni's ability to stimulate the production and activity of various defense substances to directly "attack" cancer. Over the last several years, a relatively small yet impressive body of research has focused on noni and cancer. One of the first key studies, which was presented at the 83rd Annual Meeting of the American Association for Cancer Research in 1992, dealt with the antitumor activity of noni used on mice suffering from Lewis lung carcinoma.

Anne Hirazumi, Ph.D., considered by many to be one of today's top noni researchers, led a team from the University of Hawaii in a thorough testing of noni and its touted cancer-fighting abilities in cell and animal models. Initially, Dr. Hirazumi's team treated cancerous lung cells with a polysaccharide-rich noni preparation. This did not significantly affect the cancer cells. However, upon introducing peritoneal exudate cells (PEC), model cells for immune function, to the mix of cancerous cells and noni preparation, the PEC defense cells were activated. These cells proceeded to kill a large number of the cancerous cells, ultimately resulting in a significant reduction in tumor growth.

To further test noni's ability to encourage the immunological strengthening response against cancerous cells, the researchers administered different types of noni preparations to mice with Lewis lung cancer, and withheld the noni from a control group with cancer. The results of this portion of the study were indeed impressive. The first group, consisting of 78 mice, was given crude noni juice. A second group, considered the control group, was not given noni juice. Of the 55 mice not treated with the juice, not one was cured (or lived longer than 50 days). However, of the 78 mice given the noni juice, 20 mice were cured. Additionally, their survival rates were substantially longer than the untreated mice. In fact, they were up to 119 percent longer, more than twice as long!

The second experiment, consisting of a control group of 58 and a group of 61 given a noni precipitate (a more concentrated preparation of noni juice), provided similar results. In the control group, not one was cured. However, of the noni-fed group, 20 were cured (which constitutes a 32 percent cure rate). Consequently, and not surprisingly, the survival rates were significantly higher for the noni group—up to 118 percent higher! How did noni produce such an effect in these mice? As pointed out previously, one of the specific goals of this study was to see if noni could stimulate the function of the immune system. Preliminary testing showed that the noni preparation did indeed invigorate the potential anticancer activity of PEC cells, suggesting the strong possibility of noni's ability to strengthen the body's immune system.

In later testing, Hirazumi and her team conducted a series of studies to determine if noni could enhance the production of macrophages, the cells responsible for literally destroying and consuming dangerous toxins, cells and organisms. They concluded that these tests indicated that noni "could stimulate the activation of macrophages." Specifically, noni stimulated the activity of nitric oxide, tumor necrosis factor-alpha, and interleukin 1ß, all of which are recognized as anticancer agents.

The study also included the testing of noni's action with several well-known anti-cancer agents to see if the therapeutic effects of either the drugs or noni would be enhanced. Hirazumi concludes that using noni as a supplementary treatment with below-normal doses of anti-cancer drugs such as adriamycin, 5-fluorourcil (5FU) or vincristine could produce excellent benefits with lessened side effects than just the drugs alone.[1]

What do the results of this study ultimately mean? One must first consider that this trial was conducted using only cell and animal models; consequently, the findings can't be directly transferred to humans. Also, the study only tested one kind of cancer; therefore, a substantial amount of additional research is needed to conclusively verify noni's anticancer properties in animals or humans.

However, despite the cautious attitude that we must take with a study such as this, the results do offer exciting possibilities for the prevention and treatment of cancer. The fact that noni's ingredients can directly impel the body's defense forces to act against proliferating cancer cells is certainly worth looking at. The researchers themselves acknowledged noni's apparent ability to enhance immune function, its curative effects, and its role in improving survival time. The researchers also were supportive of noni's capacity to complement drug therapies in fighting cancer. The study's conclusion suggests "important clinical applications of noni as a supplemental agent in cancer treatment. . . ."

Another very recent study (its results are just coming out as of this writing) also supports the notion that noni can aid the body in fighting cancer. In the study, conducted by researchers at the University of Illinois College of Medicine at Rockford, one group of lab mice was given only drinking water, while another group was given a mixture of water and noni juice (consisting of only 10 percent noni juice) for one week. On the last day of the experiment, each animal in both groups was given a specific dose of DMBA, a known cancer-causing agent.

Twenty-four hours after administering the DMBA, the vital organs—the heart, liver, lung and kidneys—of the animals were examined and tested using a DNA isolation process. Here's what the examination revealed.

We know that the markers used to determine the cancer activity of a substance are called DNA adduct markers. The lower the number, the more protection one has against developing cancer. The group given noni was examined, then compared against the other group not given noni juice. In the group given noni, the quantity of these markers found in the liver were reduced by 60 percent. In the heart, they were reduced by 75 percent. There was a 70 percent reduction in the lungs and a 90 percent reduction in the kidneys.[2] Mian-Ying Wang, M.D., the head of the research team, found these results extremely promising. I find them exciting as well, considering that a medical doctor heading a team at a medical research school engineered the study. And in view of the results of other studies, as well as the data from my own survey, these findings are not surprising.

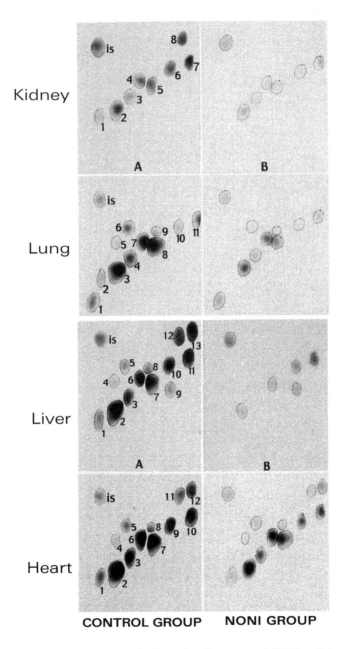

Figure 5.1: **Radiographic Density Pattern of DNA adduct markers (single nucleotide) from two-dimensional thin chromatography.** *In simple terms, the markers on the right, which are taken from the group given noni juice and which show less density, indicate more protection against cancer.*

Noni's Cancer-Fighting Agents

While noni does not contain all known cancer-fighting substances, research has revealed that it can stimulate the production, activity and effectiveness of many immune system agents, most of which are directly involved in the body's constant fight against cancer.

XERONINE

First in noni's impressive lineup is xeronine, an alkaloid both contained in small amounts in the noni fruit and formed in the body with another substance from noni, which is called proxeronine. Until the 1950s, there was little information available on either noni or its valuable compounds. Dr. Ralph Heinicke, the pioneer of noni research, first discovered the "xeronine system," and postulated that xeronine is essential to all cells to maintain normal function. As has been discussed in chapter 4, there is evidence to support the theory that xeronine and other nutrients are collected, packaged and "shipped" by the Golgi apparatus to damaged or malfunctioning cells (such as cancer cells).

NITRIC OXIDE

As outlined in chapter 4, noni extract has been shown to promote the biosynthesis of nitric oxide, a multi-talented substance whose abilities, in addition to fighting cancer, include lowering high blood pressure, fighting cardiovascular disease, and inhibiting viral and bacterial activity. Says researcher Dr. Anne Hirazumi concerning nitric oxide's role in immune function, "NO [nitric oxide] produced by activated macrophages plays a role in the host protection against pathogens as well as tumors . . . ." Dr. Hirazumi also goes on to note that NO can effectively kill pathogens by destroying the DNA synthesis of such cells and by poisoning them. As noted earlier in this book, there is considerable excitement surrounding nitric oxide and its multifaceted abilities, so much so that researchers investigating its health benefits won the Nobel prize for medicine in 1998.

INTERLEUKINS

There are several interleukins thought to be stimulated by the consumption of noni. Like most of the cells that aid the immune system in its fight to keep the body safe, interleukins are multifaceted. In general terms, interleukins are hormones that carry messages from one immune cell to another, informing the receiving cell to speed up its multiplication when there is danger of invading pathogens. Interleukins also enhance the production of B-cell antibodies and promote the cytotoxicity of NK cells. They also can play a role in activating T lymphocytes. Other research indicates that interleukin-4 has a direct inhibitory effect on the growth of tumor cells, and when acting with interleukin-2, it enhances the production of T-lymphocytes. Other interleukins, like interleukin-10, have the potential to be used as anti-inflammatory agents for chronic inflammations or autoimmune disorders such as Type 1 diabetes, multiple sclerosis and rheumatoid arthritis.[3]

INTERFERON

The type of interferon which is stimulated by noni, interferon-y, was originally thought of as a viral inhibitor. However, its major biological effects are now recognized as aiding the activation of macrophages and the overall process of cell-mediated immunity. Interferon is a multitalented player for the immune team. According to Dr. Hirazumi:

> [Interferon] activates the cytotoxicity of macrophages against tumor cells and microbial pathogens, acts synergistically with other agents, such as lipopolysaccharide, to induce the macrophage production of IL-1B [interleukin 1B], TNF-a [tumor necrosis factor-a] and NO [nitric oxide] and enhances the antigen processing and presentation by macrophages . . . IFN-y has a stimulatory effect on the proliferation of Th1 (thymus) cells and an inhibitory effect on the proliferation of Th2 cells [both thymus cells]. It augments CTL [T-cells] and NK [natural killer cells] cytotoxicity, while inhibiting B cell activation and the effects of IL-4 [interleukin-4] production.[4]

TUMOR NECROSIS FACTOR

Tumor necrosis factor (TNF) is a substance secreted by various macrophages (stimulated by noni) to kill tumor cells. The primary secretion of macrophages, TNF has been found to play a principal role in inflammation and immune response. It is also able to stimulate the growth of blood vessels, and because of this, is involved in the healing of wounds.

LIPOPOLYSACCHARIDE (LPS)

The outer layer of the membrane that encloses certain bacteria is composed mainly of LPS. Found nearly everywhere in the environment, LPS may actually play a role in the development of our immune system. Typically, the presence of LPS in the bloodstream signals the presence of gram negative bacteria, and the components of the immune system circulating in the bloodstream respond to it in a manner that eliminates the invading organism. It has been shown to encourage the synthesis and the release of cancer fighting substances such as tumor necrosis factor-a and interleukin-1. LPS production is also stimulated by noni.

NATURAL KILLER CELLS

Natural killer cells, whose production is also stimulated by the presence of noni, are the immune system's "green beret" cells. This lymphocyte is not very picky about what it will or won't kill, and can recognize virally infected cells as well as some tumor cells. Needless to say, they are very effective in ridding the body of such cells.

My Survey: Noni and Cancer

From a medical standpoint, it is quite evident that cancer is a topic that draws a lot of attention, both from patients and their doctors. I would certainly include myself in this group. Needless to say, then, I was very intrigued by the overwhelmingly positive feedback I received from the more than 900 individuals who were taking noni to help with their cancer treatment. In fact, nearly two thirds (65 percent) reported that supplementation with noni helped lessen the severity of either cancer symptoms or of side effects associated with their current treatment (such as chemotherapy). There are a wide variety of reports. Some patients have stated that noni helped diminish the severity of pain. Others report that it helps minimize nausea related to standard chemotherapy or radiation therapy. Others say that it has helped them regain their appetite as well as to regain normality in their digestion and elimination processes. The rest of this chapter provides some intriguing and possible explanations as to how noni achieves these results.

"Energy Balance" and Cancer: The Link

Over the course of the last several years, it has come to light that cancer has a very strong link with the body's energy. Energy plays a crucial role in every process involved in keeping the human body alive. Without energy there is no growth and no cell replication—without energy there can also be no life. So a key to optimal health is what is generally known as energy balance.

For human beings, the negotiable currency of energy comes mainly in the forms of glucose and triglycerides. These we calculate in calories, which are a measure of heat. Each of us must burn a certain number of calories in order to maintain our basal metabolic rate, or BMR, which are those necessary functions of breathing, circulation, digestion, and so on that keep us alive. And so that means we must burn, and thus have stored or consumed, a minimum number of calories per day.

If calories were all we needed—the way a car needs only gasoline— the dietary considerations of life would indeed be easy. But even a car needs more than gasoline—otherwise there would be no need for mechanics. Just like a car, our bodies need a certain level of preventa-

Noni and Cancer: Diana's Story

"Two days before Christmas 1994, I heard the words that every woman fears: 'From all indications, it appears you have breast cancer.' My doctor, a wonderful young man, told me that directly following the holiday, I would need a biopsy to be sure. I don't need to tell you that Christmas was not a happy time that year. As expected, the biopsy showed that I indeed had breast cancer. Further testing revealed it had spread to my lymph nodes. I immediately underwent a lumpectomy and began chemotherapy. It was a difficult time and yes, all of my hair fell out. My only consolation was that I did not have to experience the added trauma of losing my breast.

"During this time, I began suffering from depression, so much so that I was given a prescription for Zoloft to help alleviate the problem. Nearly two years later, after much suffering and an outlook that was not very good, I was introduced to noni. Intrigued, I began taking it, figuring I had nothing to lose. After only a couple weeks, I noticed that I felt generally better. After about two months, however, I realized that it was the noni that was making the difference.

"Since then (it's been over two years), my improvement has been dramatic. My doctors are amazed at how far I have come: my blood count has returned to completely normal, my energy levels are as high as before the cancer, and my depression has basically disappeared (I went off Zoloft soon after beginning on the noni, and have never felt the need to go back on). Despite the fear that the cancer could come back, I am now just a few short months away from that infamous five-year mark. And every day of cancer-free living is one more step away from that fear. Needless to say, I plan to take noni for the rest of my life!"

tive maintenance. Your physician can help you with some of this maintenance, and you'll do some of it consciously (like brushing your teeth, exercising, and choosing your foods wisely). But most of it your body accomplishes on its own, provided you keep it supplied with the materials to do so. In this regard, physical activity and nutrition are the primary tools your body needs to keep up these functions.

Energy, like many things in life, needs to be in balance in order for bodily systems to work properly. Overfill your gas tank or put in too much oil, and you not only have a mess, but you can also seriously damage your car. However the process of metabolism is more complex than just fueling up and burning the fuel. The word metabolism itself derives from the Greek meaning "to change shape," and that's exactly what metabolism is about, not only the transformation of raw fuel into usable forms of energy, but also the expulsion of waste products created by the burning of fuel. When we eat, our bodies take the basic elements of food—the macronutrients of protein, carbohydrate, fat, and others—and transform them into forms of fuel our bodies can use. That fuel is then converted into energy by the cells. Metabolism consists on one level of the processing of raw energy (eating, digestion, combustion, and exhaust) and on another level, of cellular "housekeeping." And it requires more than just calories to keep these interlocking and intertwined systems working—otherwise we could just eat candy bars all day.

In addition to the minimum amount of calories we need to maintain basic metabolism, each of us needs an additional but variable amount of energy to accomplish all of our daily physical tasks. For instance, a roofer who is constantly lugging heavy shingles up ladders and working in the hot sun has considerably different energy needs than someone who works sitting at a computer terminal.

Here's a pretty simple formula for energy balance: The average number of calories consumed minus the average number of calories burned equals your energy balance. We should exist in energy equilibrium, burning on average the same amount we consume. An increasing number of us, however, live with a positive energy balance, meaning that we consume more than we burn. And in this case, a positive is really a negative. What happens to the excess? The body stores it, usually as fat.

Ideally, after reaching our full growth, we would maintain energy equilibrium. This doesn't necessarily mean we'd eat and burn the same number of calories every day. It means that over a given period of time, say between one and three weeks, the calories we consume would roughly equal the calories we burn.

Energy excess has been linked to cancers across the board. In several comprehensive studies, women who had the lowest risk for cancer had body weights ranging from 20 percent below average to 10 percent above. Obese women, defined as more than 40 percent overweight, were found to have a whopping 55 percent increased likelihood of dying from cancer over women of average weight. Obese men were found to have a 33 percent greater likelihood of dying from cancer than those of average weight. Lowest incidence among men was also found in body weights 20 percent below average to 10 percent above.

ENERGY RESTRICTION AND CANCER PREVENTION

The evidence indicates that if a body's energy supply is in equilibrium, if the body has a healthy ratio of fat to lean body mass (the body is fit and in the range mentioned above), and if the body's cells have adequate nutritional assistance to keep their natural, built-in defenses in top working order, then the energy we consume will be used by the body's normal tissues and processes. Cancer will, more often than not, stop before it starts. A key part of this equation is physical activity, the only reliable way to maintain that healthy ratio of fat to lean body mass.

When the body is in a state of energy equilibrium, mutant cells that slip past the body's guard won't have as much energy available to develop. Energy equilibrium, then, is one of the most important aspects of stopping cancer before it starts. But animal studies, as well as some human research, have also shown possibilities that restricting energy, whether through exercise, careful eating habits, or both, can seriously inhibit or halt cancer cell proliferation.

Why? Well, we're not exactly sure. It is possible that energy intake controls cell growth. Metabolism is, from one aspect, the turnover of cells. The availability of excess energy may increase cell replication and thus cancer risk. In other words, the more times a cell replicates, the more opportunities there are for the reproduction of that cell to go awry. It is also very possible that obesity makes for higher levels of chemical carcinogens stored in body fat. Excess energy may also lead

"What A Blessing Noni Is!"

Betty explains the effect noni juice had on a large, abnormal growth in her breast:

"Three years ago, I had a mammogram showing a small shadow and what my doctor called a 'thickening in the breast.' Shortly after, I had another mammogram that indicated this 'thickening' was now a growth of five and a half centimeters. I was told to get a biopsy immediately; however, I chose to wait until after Thanksgiving as we were going out of town to visit family.

"Before we left, a friend offered me a bottle of Tahitian Noni Juice™ and suggested hopefully that if I took it, I would see some benefit. I began taking the noni juice, and within three weeks, had consumed about a bottle and a half.

"After our trip was complete, I immediately went in for the biopsy. The surgeon felt for the lump, but could not find anything. Another mammogram was immediately taken, which yielded no trace of the growth. They sent me to another hospital in Springfield, Missouri, where three more mammograms were taken in succession. Again, no trace of the growth could be found. The perplexed doctor proclaimed that a miracle had taken place. I certainly agree—what a blessing noni is!"

to breast cancer by modifying the turnover of hormones, some of which, after menopause, occur only in adipose or fat tissue.

Noni, Energy Levels and Cancer

This brings us to the question as to what noni has to do with the body's effective management of energy. If the body is to operate at an optimal level, every cell must function optimally, which means a proper consumption and conversion of energy. However, we all know that our bodies generally operate in a less than optimum manner, thereby deteriorating or skewing the balance of energy. As we've already discussed, noni, and specifically many of its compounds, can provide individual cells with the needed nutrients to allow "sick" or malfunctioning cells to repair themselves and perform at peak level. It is my belief, as well as that of many others, that noni can positively affect the basic function, including the metabolism and utilization of each cell in the body, thereby bringing about peak performance. One only has to hear the feedback of thousands of noni users concerning the effect of noni on energy levels. Most of these people probably consume more calories than they utilize, yet they feel that they have very little energy to perform the day's tasks. After using noni, even for a short time, the majority of these people report a significant improvement in their moods, "pep," and the energy to achieve what they want. In essence, noni seems to enhance the body's utilization of energy.

Additionally, Mona Harrison, M.D., former assistant dean of the Boston University School of Medicine, and former chief medical officer at D.C. General Hospital, believes that frequency modulations in the body's energy may account for some of noni's positive actions. Noni juice has its own specific frequency; this frequency, along with xeronine and the other compounds in noni, is what she believes enhances noni's therapeutic abilities. In the end, noni, along with proper diet and adequate exercise, can help bring the body's basic processes and functions, including that of maintaining proper energy levels, back into balance. And as we've already discussed, energy can have a profound effect on both the prevention and treatment of cancer.

Complementary Therapies to Noni

GENERAL LIFE STYLE RECOMMENDATIONS

Nutritional choices. Choose a diet that is predominantly plant-based, rich in a variety of vegetables and fruits, legumes, seeds, whole grains and foods that have been minimally processed.

Body weight. Avoid being overweight or significantly underweight (mostly a problem with elderly individuals).

Physical activity. The point is this—be active. If all of the benefits of exercise could be combined in a pill form (and I'm sure there are pills marketed as such), people would flock to this "miracle" pill. If your occupational activity is low or moderate, take an hour's break to engage in a brisk walk or something of similar intensity each day. In addition, try to engage in vigorous physical activity (where you actually sweat) for a total of at least an hour each week.

EXERCISE RECOMMENDATIONS

Imagine a new "miracle" cure that could:

• help you lower high blood pressure and high cholesterol levels.
• help you lose weight.
• help you improve your circulation.
• help you reduce your risk of cancer, cardiovascular disease, obesity, diabetes, osteoporosis, arthritis, and a host of other diseases.
• help you sleep better, improve your concentration and productivity at work, and improve your moods.
• improve your sex life and your social life.

In reality, you don't need to imagine such a miracle cure because it is real. You don't need to line up at the store, order by midnight tonight, or use your credit card to order. This miracle is not only cheap—even free—but it's also available wherever you are, whenever you want it.

What is it? Evalee Harrison, executive director of the Health and Movement Institute in Emeryville, California, tells us what "it" is: "Good old physical activity—known as exercise." She says that exercise is something that is not only extremely healthy but also something that can be very enjoyable and satisfying, just as long as you move. Many of us think we don't have time for exercise, or that it's really not that important. The reality is that most of us can work in time for exercise, and that the benefits of exercise increase in proportion to its frequency and strenuousness. If we can exercise as little as twenty minutes a day, it's like money in the bank.

Pinpointing the effects of fitness on cancer risk is not easy because people who are physically fit tend to have healthier lifestyles overall. Several studies, however, suggest that physical activity itself is critical in cancer prevention. Exercise broadly affects metabolism, but its key role in helping to prevent cancer may be the role it plays in balancing the calorie equation (which we have already discussed in this chapter). Summarized briefly, cancer is a disease largely connected with energy, and opportunistically seems to spring up more readily in obese and overweight bodies where unused energy is plentiful.

In several studies, scientists have observed that people who live sedentary lifestyles have a higher risk of developing different types of cancer than their more active counterparts. Confirming these findings, a study carried out at the Harvard School of Public Health found that women who participated in college athletics had a 35 percent lower rate of breast cancer and a 60 percent lower rate of cancers in the reproductive system in later years than those who had not been involved in athletics.

Why is this? Again, the answers aren't entirely clear, but many experts believe that people who burn more calories (as is the case with those who are regularly involved in physical activity) have an easier time maintaining an equilibrium of energy, which has been connected to cancer risk.

Where does noni fit in with an exercise regimen? It is my belief that it can enhance physical exercise because of its adaptogenic abilities. Of course, if you aren't exercising at all, this may all be a moot point. If you begin exercising regularly, however, noni will be able to help your body manage its energy stores and attain a balance of energy, a definite advantage in preventing and treating cancer.

So the choice is yours: gardening, dancing, swimming, jumping rope, karate, splitting wood, hiking, walking, washing the car, horseback riding, canoeing—the list can be nearly endless. The point is to just move, move every day, for just a few minutes each day. And using noni can only enhance the benefits experienced through physical exercise.

DIET/NUTRITION RECOMMENDATIONS

It is no secret that diet is extremely important to enjoying good health. But most of us know that today's prevalent lifestyles often make it difficult to consume an ideal diet. Thus dietary supplements—like noni—can make substantial contributions to the fulfilling of certain nutritional needs that our bodies may have.

But noni is not alone in its nutritional value. There are many things we can do to improve our dietary habits and make full use of the nutrition possibilities available to most of us. The majority of those familiar with noni would agree that noni's healthful benefits are probably enhanced by the presence of other necessary nutrients. The following should be considered in not only improving your dietary habits, but also as a way to improve noni's health-promoting action.

Fruits and vegetables. Eat 15–30 ounces (one to two pounds, or five servings) of a variety of fruits and vegetables daily all year long. If that seems like a lot, it really isn't. Fruits and vegetables are mostly water, and water is heavy. For instance, a good size pear or apple can weight in the neighborhood of half a pound, so only two similar servings of fruit, combined with two or three servings of vegetables, puts you where you want to be. Though we haven't discussed this much, there is considerable evidence that sprouts and grasses, such as wheat grass and bean sprouts, are not only nutrient rich but also high in anti-cancer compounds.

If you're wondering what types of fruits/vegetables to eat, variety is the key. But it is also very important to eat more vegetables than fruit (about a 65–35 percent ratio), with leafy, green vegetables comprising the significant portion of your vegetable intake.

Other plant foods. Eat approximately seven daily servings of a variety of the following "energy" foods: 1) cereals (but avoiding those that are highly processed), 2) legumes and peas, and 3) roots and tubers.

Alcohol. This is a drug, and an addictive one at that, which interferes with the metabolism of many nutrients. It is a potent carcinogen and a promoter of poor dietary habits. While some research indicates that red wine (which may contain cancer-fighting ingredients) could be beneficial, the risks associated with excess alcohol consumption far outweigh its potential benefits. In fact, some research suggests that women with any degree of breast cancer risk should avoid alcohol entirely.

Meat (domesticated red meat, beef, pork, and lamb). The available evidence suggests that it is best to consume very little red meat. You can obtain most of the necessary nutrients that red meat provides, such as protein and iron, from other sources. If you must eat red meat, go for the leanest cut possible. Great alternatives to red meat include fish, vegetable products like legumes and soy, skinless poultry, and game animals or birds.

Fats and oils. Limit consumption of fatty foods, particularly those of animal origin. Choose modest amounts of vegetable oils. These should be mostly polyunsaturated oils, like sunflower or soy oils, or monounsaturated oils, such as olive oil.

Salt. Try to limit consumption of salted foods and the use of extra table salt. Using herbs and spices can do wonders for adding flavor.

Preparation of food. Avoid eating charred meats. Foods that are cooked by steaming, boiling, poaching, stewing, or baking should be the preferred methods of preparation.

Tobacco. This one is simple: Avoid it entirely.

SUPPLEMENTATION

There are a host of substances—herbs, vitamins, minerals, phytohormones all fit into this category—that have anticancer benefits. Some work to prevent cancer, while others are adept at helping the cancer sufferer regain energy and experience a minimizing of symptoms. Of course, many would say that noni would fall into the category of nutritional or dietary supplement, mainly because there are few people today, even in noni's native areas, that consume it regularly as a food staple. While there is no way we could adequately discuss here the benefits of all supplements that have cancer-fighting benefits, the following is a list of the substances most recognized for their anti-cancer capabilities.

Vitamin C with bioflavonoids. While many vitamins and minerals can help fight cancer, vitamin C has been shown time and time again to be a powerful antioxidant as well as cancer fighting agent (especially when coupled with bioflavonoids). Research has shown that vitamin C plays a role in fighting cancer of the breast, stomach, pancreas, rectum, cervix, esophagus and lungs.[5]

Soy isoflavones. Also called phytoestrogens, isoflavones have the ability to block the carcinogenic effects of estrogen in breast tissue. They also inhibit activity by the enzymes that promote cancer cell growth, and can interfere with the blood vessel network necessary for a tumor to survive. Compounds found in isoflavones resemble closely the drug tamoxifen, which is used to fight breast cancer.

Beta carotene. Again, most vitamins and minerals are beneficial in helping the body retard cancerous growths, but beta carotene is especially key in helping the body fight the cancer war. It has been shown to help transform malignant cells and retard tumors.

Indole-3 carbinol. Found in cruciferous vegetables like broccoli and cabbage, these compounds have been linked to the prevention of both breast and prostate cancers.

Essential fatty acids. Though there is still research to be carried out, there is plenty of data to suggest that essential fatty acids can inhibit the growth of existing cancers and lower the risk of certain cancers.

Vitamins A and E. Both of these essential vitamins have been shown time and again to aid the body's immune systems. They can help repair tissue damaged by radiation or chemotherapy, diminish the effects of such treatments and slow the development of various types of cancer.

B-complex vitamins. There is ample research indicating that many B vitamins have a prominent role in helping the body perform the necessary functions to rid itself of cancerous cells. Vitamin B12 has been shown to help battle lung cancer, and a deficiency of vitamin B6 has been linked to the creation of certain malignant tumors.

Pau d'Arco. Very popular as a cancer fighter, there is ample evidence to show that it can indeed fight cancer and, specifically, reverse tumor growth.

Other supplements. The list could go on and on, but here are a few more worth investigating—coenzyme Q10, acidophilus, amino acids, germanium, selenium, vitamin D, spirulina/chlorella, ginseng, barberry root, calcium/magnesium combination, lycopene, shark liver oil, cat's claw, maitake, shitake and reishi mushrooms, d-glucaric acid, kelp, and garlic. (Interestingly, I wrote a book on shark liver oil, titled *Shark Liver Oil: Nature's Amazing Healer,* and now recommend that for optimal benefit, people add noni to their shark liver oil regimen.)

MISCELLANEOUS COMPLEMENTARY THERAPIES TO NONI

Seek emotional and psychological support. The will to live and be happy is paramount. There is ample evidence linking the emotional state of body and mind with the development of cancer.

Join a support group. This coincides with the above suggestion, but studies indicate that becoming involved in such a group is linked with significantly longer survival times.

Practice stress-reduction techniques. Exercise therapies involving stress reduction, such as yoga, can also play a pivotal role in the positive response to cancer.

Laugh every day. Laughter certainly is the "best" medicine.

Consider a detoxification program. Detoxification programs, which include a liver "flush" or juice fast, can aid the body in helping direct its energy towards the most menacing toxin: cancer.

Improve spirituality. Spiritual health is also important to maintaining good health. Though difficult to pin scientific explanations on how it helps, studies have made definite links with religious conviction, or a strong belief system, and the successful treatment of cancer and other diseases.

How Noni Helped Me with My Cancer

"I Felt 100 Percent Better!"

Stephen had been hospitalized for over three weeks after having surgery for colon cancer. He describes his experience with noni:

"The entire time I was in the hospital, my condition was not good. I was completely unable to tolerate any food, and had to be fed via an IV. About this time, my sister brought the doctor some information on noni, and asked if we couldn't allow for a few drops to be put under the tongue a couple times a day. The doctor agreed.

"So we began the treatment. About this time, the doctor determined that they would probably need to perform another surgery to check for a blockage in my intestines because I'd had very little movement since the surgery. After only one day of taking the noni, I began to feel some activity in my bowel region. That evening, I had a bowel movement, the first in over three weeks. The next morning, my IV was removed and I was started on a liquid diet. One day later I had a 'soft' meal and that evening a regular meal. I had regular bowel movements over those few days.

"The miracle of this experience occurred the next day, when I was discharged from the hospital to continue my recovery at home. Only a few days before I was scheduled for surgery because of a poor response to the first surgery. After only three days of taking Tahitian Noni Juice™, I felt 100 percent better. Thank God for noni!"

Chapter Summary Points

- Despite recent advancements in cancer treatment, noni offers a viable and supporting therapy to help fight cancer and lessen side effects of other treatments, such as chemotherapy.
- The body has various immune cells and substances, such as interferon, nitric oxide, and natural killer cells, that effectively seek and destroy cancerous cells.
- Two studies from researchers at American universities have resulted in very promising findings. While the studies showed noni to be effective in fighting specific cancers in animal models, these studies only support other evidence that noni can aid the body in fighting cancer.
- My survey of more than 10,000 noni users found that nearly two-thirds of those taking noni to help with their cancer experienced either a lessening of their symptoms or a lessening of side effects from other treatments such as chemotherapy.
- There are tremendous amounts of data indicating that rigorous attention to diet, dietary supplements, exercise, stress-release therapies and other therapies can have a profoundly positive impact on cancer. I also believe that if incorporated into a lifestyle of healthful habits, noni can be of great benefit for the cancer patient.

Noni and Diabetes

DIABETES. WE ALL know someone who has it, maybe a friend, maybe a family member, maybe a colleague at work. We hear about it on the news, and we know that it's often a serious disease. Some of us think it may even be deadly. But what do we really know about diabetes? The truth is, most people don't know what diabetes is, or how it really affects the human body.

The fact is, diabetes is a complex, serious and sometimes deadly disorder. It is the nation's third leading fatal disease, behind only heart disease and cancer, and kills an estimated 150,000 people in the United States alone. Diabetes is the leading cause of blindness in working-age Americans, the single leading cause of end-stage kidney failure, the leading cause of lower-extremity amputations (such as toes and feet), and a principal risk factor in the onset of heart disease and stroke. Of course, the financial costs of the disease are staggering, resulting in more than $92 billion per year in health-care costs and lost productivity. Needless to say, the emotional costs, both to those with diabetes, their families and friends, can't be measured.

But there is good news. Recent research indicates that diabetes can be controlled and its effects limited. Though there is still no "cure" for diabetes, there is every reason to have confidence and hope that a diabetic can lead a long, active, and productive life. A 10-year national study, completed in 1993, indicated that people with insulin-dependent diabetes, or Type I diabetes, were able to reduce their risk of developing serious long-term complications by 50 percent or more by keeping their blood sugar as close to normal as possible. To a large degree, this can be done simply by modifying the diet to reflect more wise and healthy choices.

Just as science has revealed how to reduce the risk of serious complications through dietary means, there are other ways to reduce this risk and improve the overall health of the diabetes sufferer. In reviewing the historical literature as well as the findings of my own research, I believe that noni can significantly help further reduce the risks of diabetes and contribute to overall improved health. But before we discuss noni's link to diabetes, it's important we understand the basics of diabetes—what it is, the causes, and symptoms—before we can understand how noni may help.

What is Diabetes?

Described in simple terms, diabetes is a disorder in the way your body turns food into energy. The problem centers around a substance called insulin, which your body uses to convert food to energy, and the process used by individual cells in utilizing that energy. Let's take a quick look at the entire process.

How The Body Normally Produces Energy

Quite simply, you can't live without food. The body needs food to nourish itself and sustain life. Food provides both fuel and building material for the body. It produces energy, builds and repairs body tissue, and regulates the manifold body functions and processes. But before food is used by the cells, it has to undergo some biological "steps." First, your body must break down the food you eat into its basic ingredients. These nutrients fall into three major categories—carbohydrates, proteins, and fats.

Carbohydrates, the most abundant of nutrients, are found in most food. Often "starches" and "sugars," they are found in bread, pasta, fruits, and vegetables. Proteins are most abundantly found in meats, poultry, milk, and fish. Fats are found in such foods as vegetable oils, meat, cheese and other dairy products. All of these nutrients are digested, or broken down, in the stomach and intestines. Carbohydrates are broken down into a simple sugar called "glucose," which is absorbed through the wall of the intestines into your bloodstream. This is what is often called "blood glucose" or, more simply, just "blood sugar." As we have already mentioned, diabetes is a disorder in the way the body uses blood sugar, or glucose and also fats and protein.

The Role Of Insulin in Energy Production

Once glucose is absorbed into your bloodstream, it is transported to the body's cells to provide them with the basic unit of energy. But glucose can't simply flow into the cells by itself. Because all cells are enclosed within a thin membrane, something has to tell your cells that glucose is waiting outside. That something is insulin. It attaches on specified sites on the outside of the membrane called insulin receptors—much like a key that fits into a lock. Insulin is the "key" that unlocks the cells, allowing glucose to enter. Once inside, the glucose is metabolized, or "burned," by the cells for energy.

So exactly what is insulin? It is a hormone—a chemical messenger made in one part of the body to transmit "information" via the bloodstream to cells in other parts of the body. Because of the literally thousands of various processes your body needs to operate, the body must then produce many types of hormones. Insulin, made in an organ called the pancreas, is one of these hormones.

THE PANCREAS

The pancreas is a small gland situated below and behind the stomach. In an average adult, it weighs less than half a pound. The pancreas is shaped like a long cone lying on it's side, with the end tapering off into a "tail." Within this tapering tail are tiny bits of tissue, called the "islets of Langerhans," that are very important in the body's ability to metabolize glucose.

A normal pancreas has about 100,000 islets of Langerhans. Despite their funny sounding names, these islets are actually clusters of various types of cells, the most important of which are the beta cells. These cells are the tiny "factories" that both make insulin and store it until it is needed by the body.

In addition to producing insulin, the pancreas performs other important duties. Some cells produce hormones whose actions are quite different from insulin, such as glucagon. This hormone actually raises the blood's sugar—just the opposite function of insulin. The balancing actions of these two hormones help keep blood sugar in normal range, approximately 60-140 milligrams (mg) of sugar per deciliter (dl) of blood. Other pancreatic cells produce various enzymes, which aid the digestion process by "splitting" large food particles into more simple substances, which can then be absorbed through the intestinal wall into the bloodstream.

HOW INSULIN WORKS

During normal digestion, enzymes in the mouth, stomach and intestines act upon the consumed foods, breaking them down again and again (from carbohydrates, proteins and fats), finally forming them into simple substances, which enter the bloodstream in the following forms:

- Carbohydrates are converted into glucose, which is metabolized or "burned" for quick energy.
- Proteins are converted into amino acids, which provide the basic building blocks for bone, muscle, and other tissue. Proteins also can be burned for energy.
- Fats become fatty acids, which are burned for energy or stored as body fat for potential later use.

Insulin plays a vital role in the burning and storage of all these nutrients. In diabetes, however, its principal role is related to the action of glucose, the simplified form of carbohydrates. Though somewhat simple at first glance, this process is actually complex and amazing. The key players are the beta cells, whose primary responsibility is to make and store the insulin. When the beta cells sense the level of glucose rising in the blood, they respond by releasing just the right amount of insulin into the bloodstream.

As the beta cells first sense a rise in the blood sugar, they release the insulin held in storage. But many times, the body may need even more—this often happens right after a large meal, and as the blood glucose levels increase, a second stage of insulin production begins. The "control centers" of the beta cells trigger them to make even more insulin. As we have mentioned earlier, when functioning normally, the beta cells release just enough insulin to maintain blood glucose levels within the normal range of 60-140 mg/dl. And once in the bloodstream, the insulin allows the glucose to enter your body's cells to use for energy.

There's a bit more to understanding how glucose functions in the body. When you eat, you generally won't need to use all the glucose from your food immediately. So, the body takes some of the glucose and stores it for future need. Later, with the help of insulin, this extra glucose is taken up by the liver cells and changed to a form called "glycogen." Glycogen comes in handy when your body immediately needs extra energy: like during exercise, for example. At these times, your body tries to compensate by quickly changing the stored glycogen back into glucose. In addition, glycogen takes care of your overnight energy needs, a time when you normally aren't eating. Insulin also helps convert some of the extra glucose into fat, which is stored in the body's fat cells.

What Causes Diabetes?

So now that we understand a little of how the body produces energy to keep itself alive, let's look into exactly how diabetes comes about. In simple terms, diabetes is caused by a breakdown in the normal processes previously described. This can occur in one of two ways: (1) the body produces little or no insulin; or (2) though enough insulin is

produced in the body, it can't link with the body's cells. Type I diabetes, or insulin-dependent diabetes, is the result of the first defect;
Type II diabetes, called insulin resistant diabetes, is the result of the
second. It is important to note, however, that there are some similari-
ties between Type I and Type II diabetes, and that some people display characteristics of both types.

Type I: Insulin-Dependent Diabetes

Of all people with diabetes, only five to ten percent have Type I,
which develops most often in children and young adults. That's why it
was once called "juvenile-onset" diabetes. However, this type of diabetes can occur in people of any age: thus, we use the term "insulin-
dependent" diabetes to describe it.

THE PROBLEM

Type I diabetes occurs when the pancreas produces very little, or no
insulin. In short, the beta cells cease to function. Individuals who
develop Type I diabetes are insulin-dependent. What this means is
that they generally must have a daily dose of insulin from an outside
source to be able to make use of the food they consume. If they don't,
they will cease to function and survive. Usually, insulin is taken by
injection with a syringe or with a pump.

THE SYMPTOMS

By understanding what happens when the body lacks insulin, you
can understand the various symptoms of diabetes—the outward signs
that something is wrong. This is what happened to Laura. In her early
teen years, she noticed that she constantly felt tired. Usually a very
active child, she showed signs of constant fatigue—she did not want to
be involved in extracurricular activities at school or continue playing
with her school volleyball team. She also became depressed, and lost

weight despite her already slim build. It was only after she began uri-
nating numerous times every day and complaining of excessive thirst
that her mother took her to the doctor. After hearing about her symptoms and a few preliminary tests, the doctor decided that in all prob-
ability, Laura had Type I diabetes.

What are the primary symptoms of diabetes? The following list
gives a comprehensive overview of things to look for if you suspect you
or someone else has diabetes:

Lack of energy. This occurs because your body has little or no insulin
to enable your cells to change blood sugar into energy. Without energy, you feel tired.

Constant hunger. When you are unable to get energy from the sugar
in your blood, your body sends out hunger signals for more food. Of
course, a lack of sugar isn't the real problem. The problem is that your
body can't use the sugar already there.

Weight loss. This symptom often occurs because the body, unable to
use sugar in the blood as a source of energy, turns to its fat reserves for
energy. As fat is used up, you lose weight.

Frequent urination and excessive thirst. These symptoms are
caused by a condition called hyperglycemia, or high blood sugar. In all
people, whether they have diabetes or not, the blood circulates
through the kidneys. The kidneys remove waste materials from the
blood, expelling them in the urine. They also act like a "dam" to retain
important nutrients, sending them back to the blood. In the case of
diabetes, blood sugar rises to excessively high levels, which over-
whelms the kidneys. They can't send all the sugar back into circulation,
so it overflows over the "dam" into the urine. Something else accom-
panies this overflow—water, which of course results in large amounts
of urine. Consequently, as you lose fluids, you begin to feel extra
thirsty, your body's signal to take in more fluids.

Blurred vision. One consequence of having diabetes is that of sugar

"After Only Two Days of Treatment, the Wound Healed!"

Jim R., a banker suffering from Type II diabetes, reports some dramatic and amazing results after using noni. Like most diabetics, Jim suffered from various conditions as a result of the diabetes. But in his case, noni displayed its powerful adaptogenic properties. He explains:

"Because of my diabetes, I had an open ulcer for over two months that would not heal. I began taking noni juice for just general purposes. To my surprise, after only two days of treatment, the wound had healed! But it doesn't end there. I've also had a festering sore on my toe for some time. After only four days of taking noni, the sore cleared up. And the purple coloring that I've had in my leg has faded to a nice, healthy pink shade. Finally, like many diabetics, I require insulin shots. Before having started taking noni, I was taking about 120 units with every injection. Since beginning on the noni juice, the required amount has dropped to only 40 units!"

buildup in your eyes. The excess sugar draws water with it, causing the eye's outer lens to swell and ultimately distorted vision.

Other symptoms. Diabetes sufferers may experience a number of other symptoms before being diagnosed with the disorder. These may include nausea, vomiting, abdominal pain, weakness, or rapid shallow breathing. Some may even experience a diabetic coma before realizing they have diabetes.

THE CAUSE

Type I diabetes results from the destruction or damage of the beta cells in the pancreas. Why does this occur? Research has brought us closer to an answer. As yet, scientists don't know for certain, but they believe that most cases are a result of a malfunction in the body's endocrine and immune system. As we've already discussed, the main job of your immune system is to fight diseases by producing various types of cells that eliminate foreign invaders like bacteria and viruses. In certain cases, however, the immune system turns against the body and destroys the body's own cells. So, by mistake, the body destroys the pancreas' beta cells, the very cells it needs to produce insulin.

New tests now make it possible to detect faulty immune antibodies in the blood—several years before a person shows any of the common symptoms of diabetes. In adults, the destructive antibodies may be in the blood five or more years before symptoms appear. This suggests that the destruction of the beta cells doesn't occur abruptly. Instead, it is a gradual process, taking place during what is commonly called the "prediabetic stage."

This prediabetic state can be found in association with other endocrine diseases, such as thyroid and adrenal insufficiency, also called "Schmidt's syndrome." In 1965, while on the faculty of Medicine at the Johns Hopkins Medical School, I researched this problem with three medical "giants." They were Dr. A.M. Harvey, who was chairman and professor of the Department of Medicine; Dr. John L. Bennett, who was professor and chairman of the Department of Pathology; and Charles C. Carpenter, the Chief Medical Osler Service Resident at the Johns Hopkins Hospital.

Our team found that many patients with Schmidt's syndrome had not only antibodies targeted against the adrenal and thyroid glands, but also against the insulin-producing cells in the pancreas as well.

We were recognized as the first to publish that interrelationship between antibodies and the adrenal, thyroid and pancreas glands in the medical literature.[1]

Type II: Non-Insulin-Dependent Diabetes

Type II diabetes is the most common kind of diabetes, accounting for approximately 90 percent of all cases. Until recently, Type II diabetes was generally referred to as "maturity-onset" diabetes because it occurs most often in adults 40 years of age or older.

THE PROBLEM

If you have Type II diabetes, your beta cells can still produce insulin, though generally at a reduced rate, or produce "counterfeit insulin." This type of insulin is a bogus form with very little biological activity. These Type II diabetics have an increased amount of insulin, but most of it is essentially worthless.

Our Johns Hopkins Medical research team also found pancreatic antibodies in these patients. In most of such cases, there simply is not enough biologically active insulin to meet the present needs of your body. In addition, your body's cells can't respond properly to the available insulin to let the glucose in. People with Type II diabetes usually do not depend on insulin injections to keep basic functions going (though this doesn't mean that they'll necessarily have good health). That's why it is now often called non-insulin dependent diabetes. However, it's important to note that some people with this type of diabetes may still need daily injections of insulin to maintain good health.

THE SYMPTOMS

A number of symptoms are associated with Type II diabetes, which in many ways are similar to those found with Type I diabetes. However, some of these symptoms may be more subtle in their appearance, thereby making it more difficult for the average person to determine that he/she has Type II diabetes. This is what occurred with Harold. For years, he suffered from a variety of problems—he usually felt pretty "blah," his eyesight often became blurred, he often developed colds and flu (and had a hard time fighting them off), and he increasingly experienced pain in his legs during the night. Harold also felt more hungry during the day, and drank more water than he had in years. After finally going to his health care provider and undergoing a few simple tests, Harold was informed that he had Type II diabetes.

The following are the most common symptoms associated with Type II diabetes. Again, many are similar to those of Type I diabetes, though many are not as severe and/or are more gradual in their appearance.

Lack of energy. As with Type I diabetes, when your body's cells can't properly utilize the sugar available in the blood, they obviously fall short in their production of energy, and this leads to fatigue.

Increased hunger. Because the body is unable to use the available sugar for energy, it sends out hunger signals that it needs more food—what you perceive as hunger pangs.

Hyperglycemia. If the body is unable to use the glucose in the bloodstream, it starts to become backed up. When there is enough accumulated blood sugar, it creates a condition called hyperglycemia, which is high blood sugar.

Weight gain/loss. In most cases of Type II diabetes, the high levels of unused insulin increases the conversion of sugar to fat, which causes weight gain. However, there is a small percentage of Type II diabetics who actually experience weight loss.

Frequent urination and excessive thirst. These are also symptoms common to Type I diabetes. The circulating blood travels through the kidneys, where normally the unused sugar is recycled for later use or for storage. However, when the levels of blood sugar are unusually high, the kidneys are unable to recycle it all, so the excess sugar spills into the urine, drawing additional water with it and resulting in large volumes of urine. This accounts for frequent urination. Additionally, because it becomes depleted of its normal amount of fluids, your body becomes thirsty and sends out signals to tell you so.

Blurred vision. High blood sugar can lead to a buildup of sugar in the eye fluids. The excess sugar draws water with it, causing the eye's outer lens to change its shape, which, of course, distorts your vision.

Suppression of the immune system. Conditions such as infections and slow healing often signal the onset of Type II diabetes. When blood sugar is high, it is very difficult for the immune systems to function effectively. This, of course, slows the healing process, allowing

viruses, bacteria, fungus and yeast, which your body can usually overcome in a relatively short time, to linger on indefinitely. In women
with Type II diabetes, a suppressed immune system can lead to constant vaginal infections by fungi or bacteria, causing severe vaginal
itching and a general uncomfortable feeling.

Nerve irritation and damage. Also brought about by high blood
sugar, an early sign of this problem can be intermittent leg pains during the night. If this condition is allowed to continue, a serious complication called neuropathy may develop.

Other symptoms. Problems with sexual functions are reported by
men and women in both Type 1 and Type II diabetes. Men with diabetes are susceptible to impotence, the inability to achieve or maintain
an erection, because high blood glucose can both damage the nerves
controlling the flow of blood into the penis and damage the blood vessels themselves. Women may experience sexual problems as well.
Although little is known about this complication, high blood glucose
levels can cause changes or a decrease in vaginal lubrication, making
intimacy painful and less enjoyable.

There are other symptoms, some direct, some indirect, that may signal the onset of either Type I or Type II diabetes. Some people may discover that mood changes develop. For instance, you may feel less enthusiasm in your day-to-day activities. In reality, such mood changes are
probably not caused directly by diabetes. It's more likely that the gradual loss of energy, along with the other symptoms of diabetes, may cause
some people to feel unwell, which, in turn, affects their outlook on life.

THE CAUSE

The cause of Type II diabetes remains somewhat of a mystery.
However, there is some progress in pinpointing exactly what makes
the body less receptive to available blood sugar. Additionally,
researchers have determined that there probably is no single cause.
Instead, the condition seems to be brought on by a number of factors
which interact in complex ways and vary from individual to individual.

Insulin resistance. Insulin resistance occurs when the body "resists" taking sugar into its cells. This may happen because: (1) the insulin can't link with the receptors on the surfaces of cells because there aren't enough receptors; or (2) something goes wrong in the chemical reaction at the time of linking. In either situation, the body can't use the sugar in the blood and high blood sugar develops, bringing on the symptoms of diabetes.

Defect in the beta cells. In a normal pancreas, the beta cells release the right amount and type of insulin at the proper rate. After a meal, the surge of blood sugar is usually very rapid, and once some of the sugar has been used for the body's immediate needs, the rest is stored as glycogen or fat. The rate at which insulin is released then begins to decrease, keeping blood sugar levels in the normal range of 60-140 mg/dl.

The beta cells of people with Type II diabetes are often able to secrete large amounts of insulin into the bloodstream, but for some reason these cells can't respond quickly to the rising levels of glucose, such as what occurs after a meal. One probable reason is that this insulin is the "counterfeit" form. This results in a delay in the release of insulin, and by the time the beta cells get around to the job, high levels of sugar may have already accumulated in the blood.

Reduced number of beta cells. One way to remedy the "delayed-action" situation is for beta cells to produce more pure insulin. In theory, the additional insulin would take care of the excess sugar that accumulated during the delay. However, people with Type II diabetes often have fewer normally functioning beta cells, and even though these beta cells can make insulin, they generally can't make enough "good" insulin to handle the excess blood sugar caused by the delay.

Noni and Diabetes

Of the health conditions reported to be helped by noni, diabetes is one of the most common. The historical reports of the island cultures

that widely used noni for its medicinal and health promoting properties usually do not refer to diabetes by name. This is probably because
these cultures did not know that such a condition existed. However,
there are numerous reports of noni helping with symptoms and conditions that accompany both types of diabetes. For instance, noni was
commonly reported by the Kahunas with whom I and others have
talked to have helped with vision problems, the healing of lingering
infections and wounds (signs of a depressed immune system), and to
increase energy levels. These are all common symptoms of a diabetic
condition.

In addition, there are literally thousands of present-day reports that
noni can indeed help relieve the diabetic condition. While I was
amassing the data submitted by over 50 doctors and health professionals and 10,000 of their patients and clients, I was extremely surprised to learn how many individuals were taking noni to help with
their diabetes, and the high success rate these people achieved in
relieving the varying symptoms of diabetes. Specifically, more than
2,770 people decided to try using noni to treat their diabetes (most of
these were of the Type II variety); as of this writing, close to 84 percent of these reported that noni really did help relieve the symptoms
associated with their condition.

This means that over 2,325 people suffering from high blood sugar
levels, constant fatigue and blurred vision experienced significant
relief after taking noni. These same people could also have been experiencing depression, poor circulation in their toes and feet, unwanted
weight gain or weight loss, and problems with their sex lives. But soon
after supplementing with noni, the vast majority of these people saw
these symptoms reduced, or in some cases, entirely disappear. As this
chapter discusses, diabetes (particularly Type II diabetes) is a condition that can be slow in developing. Therefore, the symptoms that otherwise would indicate the condition is developing can go unnoticed or
ignored for a long period of time. Often, other conditions, such as
hyperglycemia and hypoglycemia, may be eventually linked with a diabetic condition. So, many of the people in my survey taking noni for
conditions such as vision problems may actually have had diabetes
without knowing it.

How Noni Relieves Diabetic Symptoms

As I have stated numerous times, the purpose of this book is to demonstrate how noni, when part of a holistic health plan, can enhance the body's ability to fight disease and improve health. This is the case with diabetes. Though there is no substantial research revealing exactly how noni can alleviate the debilitating effects of diabetes, there is little doubt that it does. As mentioned previously, my survey of more than 10,000 noni users indicated that diabetes was one of the conditions for which noni was most commonly used, and that more than 83 percent of the 2,773 using it experienced significant relief of their diabetic condition. There are also literally thousands of other testimonials from doctors, health professionals, and patients that attest to noni's ability to fight diabetes and regulate high blood sugar. Historical use also indicates that noni has long been used as a folk remedy for treating the various symptoms of both types of diabetes, from depressed immune function to fatigue to vision problems.

There are some entirely plausible theories behind noni's mode of action in relieving diabetes, especially of the Type II variety. First, as we covered briefly earlier in this chapter, it appears from our research at Johns Hopkins Hospital that one reason the beta cells start to fail in their performance is due to some sort of autoimmune disorder or to one or more various infections. A well-tuned immune system typically uses many different cells to carry out the numerous immune functions. These cells are in charge of identifying, killing and effectively cleaning invading pathogens from the body. However, in the case of autoimmune disorders, the immune system's defense cells turn against the body, attacking perfectly healthy and normally functioning cells.

Our research has shown that this is commonly the case with the pancreas' beta cells. This can cause a complete obliteration of the beta cells, which results in a virtual lack of insulin and the development of Type I diabetes. Or, it may lead to a lower number of functioning beta cells, which reduces the amount and purity of insulin the body can produce, and ultimately a diagnosis of a Type II diabetic condition.

This is the point where I believe that noni comes in. Current studies have revealed that noni has a potent strengthening effect on the immune system, both in enhancing the effect of already functioning immune processes and in stimulating a sluggish immune system. There are a variety of autoimmune disorders that are not well understood or are a total mystery to the medical world. For instance, lupus, fibromyalgia and chronic fatigue syndrome are all "diseases" whose causes and effects defy precise understanding by doctors and other medical professionals. Yet it is known that these and other conditions are accompanied by a dysfunctioning immune system, resulting in inflammation, pain and overall discomfort of the joints and other areas of the body. It is quite possible that the beta cells of the pancreas also suffer from the attacking defense cells of the body's immune system in the midst of one of these conditions.

It is also possible that the body's beta cells, while not completely rendered useless, are operating at only a portion of their capability. As we discussed in chapter 4, there is strong data suggesting that noni wields an adaptogenic, or normalizing, effect that can aid "sick" cells in their reparative process and thereby improve the overall performance of the corresponding tissue or organ. This could apply either to (1) malfunctioning beta cells not producing enough insulin, or (2) to the cells unsuccessfully trying to "receive" the glucose in the blood due to their reduced inability to accept insulin at its appropriate receptor site; or (3) too much biologically inactive insulin being produced. Consequently, in the case of a Type II diabetic who just can't get his or her blood sugar levels down to a safe level, noni may help repair damaged beta cells, which would result in a greater amount of insulin produced. This would ultimately lead to a more efficient conversion of the body's glucose, a more normal blood-glucose reading, and a significant feeling of well-being and overall health.

This is exactly what happened to Joyce's husband, who finally began taking noni after a friend of theirs explained how noni could help him with his diabetes. Joyce explains that "despite his best efforts to take his diabetic medication and keep to a good diet, he could not get his blood-sugar levels down below 165 mg/dl (normal is 60-140 mg/dl). However, after taking noni juice for a few short weeks, his glucose levels dropped to a very healthy 100, and sometimes even lower! I'm so thankful for being introduced to this miracle plant!"

"Other Good Things Continued to Happen!"

Timothy B., a long-time diabetic, describes the incredible success he has enjoyed using noni to treat his diabetes and other conditions.

"I am a seventy-four year-old who has had diabetes for more than 30 years. Of course, I have experienced the usual problems that come with diabetes.

"Several years ago, I had two back operations within a six-month period. The problems that necessitated the second operation seriously weakened the muscles in my right leg. After that operation, I began walking with a walker. I eventually graduated to a cane and was able to limp around without the cane.

"About this time, I began taking one ounce of noni juice every day. Initially, I noticed little or no difference. However, this would soon change. Because of my back operations, I was forced to sleep on my side. This caused my arthritic shoulder to flare up in pain, which would wake me every couple hours. Not long after having started on the noni, I awoke one morning to the realization that I had slept the entire night on only one side and had not woken once because of pain! In addition to this, my mobility has dramatically improved, and the chronic pain that was so common has diminished to almost nothing.

"Other good things continue to happen. Foot care is very critical for diabetics. Though the pulse in my feet has been relatively strong, I have over the years been losing feeling in my feet. However, not long after starting taking the noni, I noticed that I could feel the carpet when walking barefoot, and could feel the insoles of my shoes. At the same time, leg cramps that I commonly felt during the night began to subside.

"Last, but certainly not least, noni has been wonderful in helping me maintain a healthy blood-glucose reading. After only six weeks on noni, my readings were dropping drastically. So, I adjusted my insulin intake, and take one half-ounce of noni juice before every meal. I now have my blood-glucose levels stabilized. Noni truly has been a godsend!"

Noni consumption may help alleviate diabetic symptoms in other ways. For instance, noni has been shown to stimulate the body's production of two substances—scopoletin and nitric oxide—both known to improve the body's cardiovascular function, and thereby reducing conditions that often accompany diabetes. Such conditions include vision problems, poor circulation, retinopathy, and different types of heart disease. Noni also has substantial amounts of fiber, which has a wonderful effect on high blood sugar levels and improves the body's overall digestion and energy utilization processes. (Later sections of this book will discuss fiber more in depth.)

Complementary Therapies to Noni

DIET/NUTRITION RECOMMENDATIONS

Eat a high-complex-carbohydrate, low-saturated fat, high-fiber diet. This should include plenty of raw vegetables, fruits, and vegetable juices. This will reduce the immediate need for insulin, as well as lower the level of fats in the blood. Fiber will also help temper swift surges of blood glucose. Other foods thought to help maintain healthy blood-sugar levels include berries, cheese, egg yolks, fish, garlic, soybeans and soy products, and kelp (often considered a supplement).

Eat frequent, smaller meals throughout the day. This can help reduce the immediate need for a lot of insulin and maintain a lower, more normal blood-glucose level.

Avoid simple carbohydrates. This applies especially to foods high in refined flour and sugar. These result in strong, rapid surges in blood sugar, which usually can't be handled by a diabetic's malfunctioning beta cells. However, when suffering an insulin "reaction," simple sugars can quickly counter the reaction's effects.

Acquire protein from sources such as grains, legumes and other vegetables. Fish and low-fat dairy products are also acceptable sources of protein.

SUPPLEMENTATION

Chromium picolinate. There are numerous studies showing that chromium picolinate can improve the efficiency of insulin utilization, lower blood-sugar levels, reduce the need for diabetes medications, reduce obesity, and enhance the body's ability to use fat for energy.

L-carnitine, L-glutamine and taurine. These amino acids help the body reduce sugar cravings, improve its ability to produce insulin and enhance fat utilization.

Zinc, vanadium, manganese, and magnesium. All of these minerals are known to be involved in the body's maintenance of proper blood-sugar levels.

Vitamin B12. This has been shown to help prevent and even reverse some diabetic neuropathy (damage to nerves that results in sensations of numbness, tingling and pain).

Gymnema sylvestre. This Ayurvedic herb is reported to significantly lower blood-sugar levels.

Quercetin and naringin. These flavonoids can inhibit the activity of the enzyme aldose reductase, which is involved in the development of diabetic cataracts, retinopathy, and neuropathy.

Digestive enzymes. Because the pancreas also produces other substances that contribute to the proper digestion of food, taking digestive enzyme supplements can relieve stress on the body's digestive system.

Bilberry, ginkgo, pycnogenol and hawthorn. These all reportedly help protect the arteries, preventing arteriosclerosis, and slow the development of vascular problems common to diabetics, particularly in the eyes and extremities (hands, toes, fingers, etc.)

Lipoic acid. This helps prevent neuroglycosylation, the adherence of glucose to nerve endings, resulting in pain, numbness, and tingling in various areas of the body.

Essential fatty acids. Because the body is inhibited in its ability to metabolize EFAs, fatty acids such as gamma linolenic acid (GLA) and eicosapentaenoic acid (EPA) are good supplementation investments.

Fiber supplements. Even though improvements in diet can provide the added benefits of more dietary fiber, it is often helpful to add a fiber supplement to one's diet. Fiber helps maintain a more even blood-sugar level for extended periods during the day. Noni is an excellent source of fiber.

It is interesting to note that noni can act synergistically with all food and dietary supplements.

OTHER CONSIDERATIONS

Avoid stress. Stress management can play a pivotal role in the treatment of diabetes since uncontrolled and poorly managed tension and anxiety contribute to higher than normal levels of hormones, which negatively affect the actions of insulin. High stress levels can therefore contribute to elevations in blood sugar levels.

Weight management. It is no secret that reducing obesity can help relieve the various symptoms of diabetes, especially fatigue, high blood pressure and poor circulation. Of course, maintaining a proper weight helps counter the development of arteriosclerosis and other forms of heart disease, as well as a host of other debilitating diseases.

Exercise. This goes hand-in-hand with weight management. Exercise can help fight the various forms of heart disease, decrease high blood pressure, lower blood-sugar levels and cholesterol levels, and improve circulation.

How Noni Helped Me with My Diabetes

"My Blood Pressure Readings Are Completely Normal!"

Rick S. explains how noni helped him cope with his diabetic condition and its debilitating side effects:

"I have been a Type I diabetic since I was a teenager, which ultimately resulted in me needing to receive two kidney transplants. About three years ago, I began taking noni juice, and immediately felt that I had more energy. Though I needed less sleep at night, my rest was certainly satisfying. Because of the onset of neuropathy associated with my diabetes, I have not had any sensation of temperature or touch for more than 15 years. After taking the noni juice for only three days, I was able to feel the carpet and tile floors in my home, as well as the coldness in my feet from walking around barefoot.

"Because of my transplants, I've had to have regular blood work done. For the first time in 12 years, my creatinine level is now normal. All other test indicators my doctors use to monitor my health have also seen significant improvement; in fact, they're as good as they were before my transplants.

"Of course, I have other conditions related to my diabetes. One of these is high blood pressure. For years, I have been on hypertension medications to try and control it. Since beginning on the noni juice, I have been able to completely stop taking all my blood pressure medicines. I have been taking noni the entire time. My readings are now perfectly normal—120/78. I am excited to be feeling so much better and I am thankful for my amazing improvements—I believe this is entirely due to noni."

"I Did Not Need As Much Insulin!"

Gilbert R., a Type II diabetic and bilateral amputee (having lost portions of both legs), experienced incredible results with noni. He explains:

"Because I am a diabetic and amputee, I have various health challenges. Not long ago, I was approached by two friends and business associates telling me of something they were involved in—noni juice. To say the least, I was skeptical that it would work, and I was broke. But they convinced me to try it for one month, and after that time if I was not one hundred percent satisfied, I could have a full refund.

"So, I began taking it immediately. Not more than a few days later, I noticed that I did not need as much insulin! After carefully monitoring my blood sugar, I have been able to safely reduce the amount of insulin I take daily by up to 30 percent. My blood pressure is also the best it has been in years, and I have much more energy than I have had in some time.

"Another significant thing that has occurred is that my legs, which both have been amputated, do not hurt as much as they usually do. I have had an open ulcer on the bottom of my left stump for over five years that simply would not heal. Before starting the noni treatment, it had opened up to about the size of a silver dollar and was deep enough to go past the second knuckle of my index finger. I have tried numerous things to try and get it to heal. The doctor's last-ditch solution was to take an additional 12 inches off my leg—no, thank you! Since taking the noni, the ulcer has started to close and is now barely the size of a nickel. And I can barely put the end of my finger in!"

Chapter Summary Points

- Diabetes, though a serious condition, can largely be controlled through a healthful diet, careful attention to one's eating habits, a regular exercise program, and other beneficial practices.
- Despite the increase in knowledge of how to diagnose and treat diabetes, more people than ever suffer from the disease.

- Noni has long been used to treat symptoms of diabetes. My survey of noni users found that the large majority (83 percent) of those taking it to relieve symptoms associated with diabetes experienced significant benefit.

- Though it is not entirely understood how noni helps counter the effects of diabetes, I believe that it is through the xeronine system and the Golgi apparatus that malfunctioning cells (such as the insulin-producing cells in the pancreas and cells throughout the body that can't properly utilize available insulin) can once again regain at least some of their normal function. I also think that because diabetes is often linked to autoimmune dysfunction (which results in insulin-producing cells becoming damaged or destroyed), noni may improve a diabetic condition because of its ability to strengthen the immune system.

- There are literally thousands of testimonials, as well as historical data spanning hundreds of years, testifying to the notion that noni can indeed relieve the symptoms and effects of both types of diabetes.

CHAPTER

7

Noni and High
Blood Pressure

SIXTY MILLION AMERICANS have high blood pressure. The illness, commonly known as hypertension, is the most common reason people go to doctors. It's also the number one health condition for which medication is prescribed in the world today. More people are taking medication for hypertension than have ever taken medicine for any illness ever encountered in human history. It would not be a stretch to say that the occurrence of high blood pressure has reached plague proportions.

Once diagnosed with high blood pressure, you are many times more vulnerable to a host of other illnesses and ultimately premature death. For instance, those with hypertension are on average seven times more likely to suffer a stroke, four times more likely to have a heart attack, and five times more likely to die of congestive heart failure than individuals with healthy blood pressure levels.

Strictly speaking, high blood pressure is not a disease at all. It's really just an indicator of trouble in your circulatory system that results from a constellation of underlying problems affecting blood circulation. These underlying factors combine to raise blood pressure, sometimes to very dangerous levels. Yet, the disorder itself is merely a sign of underlying disease, just as fever is a sign of infection, or swelling a sign of a fractured bone.

It is important to note that high blood pressure is a condition that largely results from a Western lifestyle. It is far more common among people who live in affluent nations than it is among people of the Third World. Among citizens of "rich" nations, such as the United States, blood pressure increases with age. Close to half of Americans age 65 and older suffer from hypertension. In many Third World countries, however, blood pressure levels remain within the healthy range throughout life. The people of New Guinea and many African nations—even their senior citizens—exhibit blood pressure levels that resemble those of a healthy American teenager. Despite the fact that some racial groups of Americans suffer from higher rates of hypertension than others, it is safe to say that there is no racial immunity for high blood pressure. If you were to take those same Africans and feed them the standard American diet, you would see their blood pressures skyrocket to levels that are typical of hypertensive Americans. That is precisely the case among African Americans, 28 percent of whom suffer from high blood pressure and are consuming the ideal diet for hypertension. The disorder also attacks an estimated 16 to 18 percent of white Americans, as well as many Asians, Hispanics, Native Americans, and other ethnic groups.

If we "back up" and look at the distribution pattern of hypertension worldwide, we get a very clear picture of who suffers from the illness, who doesn't, and why. That pattern points directly at the causes of the disorder, as well as at its prevention and potential reversal. Most experts agree that high blood pressure can be reversed in a majority of cases. This can be accomplished through a diet low in fat, cholesterol, salt, and refined foods, coupled with a lifestyle that includes moderate exercise and the maintenance of normal weight. There is also ample evidence to suggest that supplementing with nutraceutical, or natural, agents—just like noni—can contribute to lowering high blood pressure through enhancing the body's ability to battle the condition. Of course, high blood pressure may accompany, or be a result of, other disorders like diabetes (which I discussed in chapter 6). In these cases as well, noni can be a valuable component of a holistic approach to reversing high blood pressure levels, thereby allowing the hypertensive individual to get off his or her medications and enjoy a healthier and more satisfying life.

Before we examine exactly how noni can help fight the effects of high blood pressure, it is important to review some important aspects of high blood pressure—its causes, symptoms and potential effects on the body.

What is Blood Pressure?

Before we define exactly what blood pressure is, let's examine how the system that carries our blood is constructed. At the core of the cardiovascular system is the heart. From the heart branch off the arteries, which are the principal pipeline for the blood carried from the heart to the various tissues and organs of the body. They are configured like a tree: the central trunk, or aorta, leaves the heart and then branches repeatedly. Eventually, the blood vessels branch into arterioles, very small vessels that are visible only under a microscope. Arterioles have muscle cells in their walls, allowing them to constrict and dilate just like the main arteries, and therefore contribute to the control and direction of blood flow to where it is most needed. The arterioles branch into even finer vessels, called capillaries, which form a delicate mesh that supplies the tissues with oxygen and other nutrients. For the blood to be able to circulate properly, a certain level of pressure is needed to force it through the arterioles and capillaries.

It's important to realize that our blood pressure is continually varying in order to meet the changing needs of our bodies. In fact, some of us have high blood pressure some of the time, and we wouldn't be able to function well if we didn't. However, only when high blood pressure is sustained for long periods of time does it become a real health concern. The changes in blood pressure were noted for real the first time that blood pressure was measured. In 1733, an English priest named Stephen Hales inserted a glass tube into a major neck artery of a horse, and was surprised to see that the blood reached a height of about eight feet in the tube. Not surprisingly, the horse didn't much enjoy having a glass tube stuck into its neck, so its ensuing struggle brought about an increase in its blood pressure, evidenced by a sharp rise of blood in the glass tube.

Defined simply, blood pressure is the force exerted on the blood as it moves through your arteries. The force of the pumping heart muscle against the resistance of the blood vessels creates the "pressure." Your blood pressure rises and falls naturally throughout the day. When you wake up, get out of bed, exercise, or experience stressful situations, your heart beats more rapidly to meet the increased demand for blood and oxygen from cells and tissues throughout the body. This increase in heart rate also increases your blood pressure during these particular times. Blood pressure falls while you rest, and especially while you sleep, because the demands on the heart are greatly diminished. In healthy people, blood pressure rises when heart rate increases, and drops into the normal ranges when the increased demand is relieved.

What the Numbers Mean

Generally, blood pressure is expressed in numbers as a fraction, such as 120/85 (read one hundred and twenty over eighty-five). Two numbers are used because there are two pressures being measured. The first pressure, called systolic, is indicated by the top number, and represents the phase when the heart contracts and pumps blood into the aorta, the body's main artery. As the blood is pushed into the arteries, they expand. The recoil of those arteries, or their contraction, creates the second type of blood pressure, called diastolic. This pressure occurs while the heart rests, the valves open, and the ventricles fill with blood. While the heart expands, the arteries contract and serve as a kind of second pumping action.

Diastolic pressure, therefore, indicates the relative flexibility of your arteries. The less flexible your arteries are the more pressure they will exert as they recoil on the blood. It's a lot easier for the heart to pump blood through soft, flexible arteries than to pump blood through hard, inflexible vessels. The degree of inflexibility of those arteries indicates how much resistance the heart must overcome to pump the blood. Naturally, the harder the vessels, the harder the heart must work.

Blood pressure is measured as millimeters of mercury (mm Hg), which dates back to a time when the original blood pressure gauges used mercury in a glass tube to indicate how high or low the blood pressure was. Originally, the blood pressure gauge indicated how much pressure was necessary to move a column of mercury up a calibrated tube. Today, the gauge, called a sphygmomanometer, or a blood pressure cuff, uses air and a spring, and the test can be performed by just about anyone at home in a few seconds. As a trained medical physician, I would urge anyone with high blood pressure, even if it is mild, to buy a cuff and check your pressure regularly at home. This will give you the most consistent and accurate reading. "Why not at the doctor's office?" you ask. Blood pressure readings are usually higher when taken at a doctor's office. This phenomenon is commonly referred to as "white-coat hypertension." Many people don't enjoy going to the doctor's office. In fact, for most it is somewhat stressful. Because of this, having your blood pressure read at the doctor's office, rather than in the comfort of your own home, will usually result in higher readings.

And regular people aren't the only ones susceptible to white-coat hypertension. It can happen even to doctors. This is exactly what happened to John McDougall, M.D.

> Recently, I went for a life insurance physical and had to have my blood pressure checked. Remarkably, I tested mildly hypertensive at 140/90. I was shocked. My blood pressure has always been excellent. How could I have high blood pressure? After the test, I drove home and had my wife, Mary, check my pressure. "If your blood pressure was any lower, you'd be dead," she said. What I had experienced was white-coat hypertension. I do not test hypertensive at home, but like many people, I test hypertensive in a doctor's office. Lots of people have this experience, so I recommend that you test your blood pressure in a setting in which you feel safe. You may not get an accurate reading, otherwise.[1]

Blood Pressure Readings: What Is Healthy?

There is no line of demarcation separating a healthy from an unhealthy blood pressure. Rather, it's a small margin in which the ranges for health and illness vary somewhat, depending on the person and other risk factors. In general, the higher the pressure, the worse the consequences. It's the same problem as trying to define when someone is fat as opposed to thin, or tall as opposed to short. Understanding this point is very important because high blood pressure is not a condition that you either have or don't have (in contrast to cancer, for example). In other words, it's a quantitative rather than qualitative disorder.

So, what is healthy? Most experts agree that a blood pressure below 140/90 mm Hg is normal, and that a pressure above 160/100 mm Hg is too high. The resulting gray area, where there is genuine disagreement among doctors, is the blood pressure area that falls between these two ranges. My own personal feeling is to keep your blood pressure below 130/85.

But a healthy reading also depends largely on the individual. Various risk factors specific to that individual can largely determine where his/her healthy blood pressure reading is. For instance, if you smoke and your blood pressure is in the gray area, then your risk of developing heart disease or a stroke, among other ailments, is certainly higher. And this is the ultimate goal—not to lower blood disease, but rather to reduce the risk of heart disease, stroke and heart attack; in other words, to keep you healthy.

Is High Blood Pressure a Disease?

Not really. Like we've mentioned before, it is usually a symptom of some other underlying condition. People with high blood pressure usually do not appear or feel sick. They function just like you and me. It's only when blood pressure gets to very high levels (malignant hypertension) that it makes people feel sick. For the majority with only "moderate" hypertension, the danger is in the wear and tear on the cardiovascular system.

Why is High Blood Pressure So Bad?

Though we've mentioned it before, it's probably worth it to explore this a little more in depth. Though everyone technically has high blood pressure some of the time, it causes problems only when it stays elevated for long periods of time. Even then, there are those who have high blood pressure who never know it, yet live long and productive lives. Unfortunately, not all are so lucky, and the reason health professionals are concerned with high blood pressure is that a definite link between it and a number of serious conditions—including strokes and heart attacks—has been established.

High blood pressure causes damage in three ways. The first is the one most think of initially—the bursting of a blood vessel. Called a stroke, this usually occurs in the brain when a small artery develops a weak spot and eventually breaks.

The second way in which hypertension inflicts damage is that it accelerates the deposition of cholesterol plaque in the arteries. This may take years to develop, but it is very difficult to detect until it causes a major blockage. These deposits can occur in the heart, causing heart attacks and angina (severe pain); the kidneys, where it causes renal failure and even higher blood pressure; the brain, where it causes strokes; and the legs, resulting in a condition known as intermittent claudication, which is pain while walking.

The final way that high blood pressure negatively affects the body is in the undue strain it puts on the heart. Because the heart has to work excessively to do its job, it grows, just like any other muscle that is used excessively. People that don't have high blood pressure, such as athletes, may also have an enlarged heart, but theirs is due to the increased amount of blood needed to accommodate their activity. People with high blood pressure, on the other hand, don't need a larger volume of blood, they simply need to push the blood they have through smaller vessels. This leads to thicker heart walls, which is bad because the heart then outgrows its own blood supply, rendering it more susceptible to the effects of plaque buildup in the arteries that supply it.

"I'll Take Noni As Long As I Live!"

Cristine, a native of Texas, is just one example of the hundreds of individuals whose lives—and cardiovascular health—have been changed because of noni. She says:

"For the past ten years, I have suffered from various health problems. First, my carotid artery has been 80 percent blocked, inoperable, with transient ischemic attacks, commonly known as 'mini-strokes.' I suffer from high blood pressure and tachycardia (excessively fast heartbeat), and I also have a benign cyst wrapped around my 7th cranial nerve. Having this cyst removed, according to my doctor, probably would result in paralysis of the entire left side of my face, including loss of taste, eye-lid control, uncontrolled drooling, and other conditions.

"Needless to say, the many medications I have been taking (and that have supposedly 'kept me alive') have produced the following side effects: extreme fatigue, blurred vision, occasional disorientation, abnormal liver enzymes, loss of apetite, diarrhea, severe headaches, bleeding gums, and others. I'd had enough!

"Not long ago, I began taking noni juice, starting with a one-ounce dose in the morning and evening, then increasing to a two-ounce dose, and now I am taking a four-ounce dose twice daily. The results have been marvelous. The 'mini-strokes' have disappeared, and I've cut my medication by 50 percent! My blood pressure has lowered to normal, and the tachycardia is gone. The cyst has significantly decreased in size! I have no more diarrhea, my headaches are gone, the bleeding gums are only a memory, and my energy levels have returned—I'll be drinking noni for the rest of my life!"

Risk Factors for Stroke and Heart Disease: The Big Three

Stroke and heart disease are the major causes of death and disability in developed countries, and there are several risk factors that make them more likely to occur. Some are things that we can't do anything about (like age and gender), but the most important are risk factors we can control. These "big three" factors—high blood pressure, smoking and high cholesterol levels—are the things that contribute most to the occurrence of heart disease and stroke. Again, if your blood pressure is somewhere close to 140/90 mm Hg, your risk of developing heart disease or suffering a heart attack and/or stroke is considered higher, especially if you smoke or have high cholesterol levels.

How Noni Helps Lower High Blood Pressure

As I was collecting the data comprising my noni survey, it soon became evident to me that noni was commonly being used to treat high blood pressure and other related conditions. Of course, this corresponded perfectly with the historical data I had collected, as well as with the information provided me by Kahunas and other traditional healers from a number of island cultures. So, I began searching the scientific data available for possible answers as to how noni could help lower hypertension.

My investigation produced a number of plausible answers. First, noni contains a substance called scopoletin, which has been scientifically proven to help constricted blood vessels dilate, thereby lowering blood pressure. Another reason noni may be able to help relieve high blood pressure is because of its stimulatory effect on the body's production of nitric oxide. As we have discussed somewhat in previous chapters, nitric oxide (NO) has been shown to have a positive effect on allowing blood vessels to be more elastic, resulting in lower blood pressure and an overall beneficial effect on the entire cardiovascular system. Finally, I believe that noni, which can enhance the body's abil-

ity to utilize the "xeronine system," provides a way for sick and damaged cells (such as those in hardened blood vessel walls) to once again
regain normal function and, consequently, lead to more healthy blood
pressure levels.

Scopoletin

A number of experts have assigned at least a portion of noni's ability to lower high blood pressure to the compound scopoletin. Though
discovered some time ago, scopoletin was only isolated from noni
extract in 1993 by researchers at the University of Hawaii. There is an
impressive body of data that reveals scopoletin's antihypertensive
properties. Despite this valuable capability, there are some who have
expressed concern over indications that scopoletin may occasionally
lower blood pressure to below-normal levels. However, in all of the
research, the thousands of case studies, and the files of user feedback
that I have reviewed, I have yet to come across one documented case
in which noni lowered blood pressure to below-normal levels.

One may ask how this is possible, seeing that noni contains scopoletin, and scopoletin has been shown to occasionally cause low blood
pressure. I believe that it is possible for a number of reasons. First, in
most botanicals that demonstrate medicinal benefits, there are a number of biochemicals, compounds, and other substances that work synergistically (enhancing each other's properties while simultaneously
preventing side effects) to create the desired health benefit. In the
case of noni, I believe this to be true.

This brings us to another explanation of how scopoletin may help
lower high blood pressure without taking it too low. Think back to the
Golgi apparatus, which we discussed in chapter 4. The role of this mini
"post office" is to package together specific amounts of various substances—hormones, biochemicals, vitamins, amino acids, fats, and other
nutrients—and "mail" them to the cells (or parts of cells) that need the
package of nutrients in order to maintain or regain normal function.
Besides scopoletin, noni contains the necessary ingredients to make

xeronine, an alkaloid that plays an integral part in promoting the synergistic activity of the various ingredients packaged in the Golgi apparatus. I believe that the scopoletin contained in noni is packaged, in just the right amount, through the Golgi apparatus, and probably teamed with xeronine to provide what eventually results in a dilation of previously constricted blood vessels and a proper blood pressure reading.

Nitric Oxide

We've already reviewed in chapter 4 what nitric oxide is, as well as its importance in the body's maintenance of a smooth-running cardiovascular system. We've also touched on some of the scientific data showing that noni stimulates the body's production of nitric oxide. While the principal study investigating noni and nitric oxide focused on NO's ability to fight cancerous cells, it is no leap of logic to assume that nitric oxide stimulated by the presence of noni extract could also be used to fight high blood pressure and contribute to an improved and healthy heart and vascular system.

So how does NO lower blood pressure? Many researchers now believe that nitric oxide may be at the core of the somewhat complex process of regulating blood pressure. Essentially, endothelium cells produce and release nitric oxide into the bloodstream, which in turn causes the smooth muscles making up the vessel walls to relax, ultimately leading to a more normal elasticity in the blood vessels, less wear and tear on the heart, and a lower, more healthy, blood pressure.

The treatment of high blood pressure with nitric oxide makes perfect theoretical sense, given the dual benefits of relaxing arteries and inhibiting blood clots. But does it really work in real patients? Hundreds of research articles suggest that the answer for many patients is a resounding "Yes!" Here are a few samplings from recently collected data:

• The study conducted by Dr. Anne Hirazumi and colleagues from the University of Hawaii clearly shows that noni extract enhances the production of nitric oxide in the endothelial cells. Though the study focused more on nitric oxide's role in fighting cancerous and other invasive organisms, the ramifications are clear. Couple this with the widespread reports that noni has a definite positive effect on high blood pressure, and it is clear that noni (and specifically, noni-induced nitric oxide) encourages the dilation of constricted blood vessels, thereby relieving hypertension and benefiting the cardiovascular system in other ways as well.[2]

• A recent clinical trial consisted of hypertensive men ranging in ages from 35 to 65 who volunteered to withdraw from blood pressure medication for one week. Each morning, they were given intravenous arginine (an amino acid known to stimulate the body's production of nitric oxide). This injection created a rapid decrease in both systolic and diastolic blood pressure in all the patients, an effect that lasted about 20 minutes. No other symptoms other than dry mouth were reported.[3]

• Another study revealed that five patients with hypertension were given intravenous arginine. They had an average high blood pressure of 154/95 mm Hg before treatment, but shortly afterwards, their systolic pressure dropped an average of nearly 30 mm Hg and the diastolic pressure decreased an average of 22 mm Hg.[4]

In addition to these scientific studies, the results of my survey—which included more than 10,000 noni juice users and 50 doctors and other health professionals—strongly support the notion that noni (through various agents and processes involving nitric oxide, scopoletin, xeronine and others) can help lower previously high blood pressure to healthy levels. As I have stated before, there is no real scientific evidence for this. But if we look at the sheer numbers of case studies, testimonials, professional opinion, and supporting data, it is clear that noni does represent an effective, safe and exciting antihypertension agent without harsh side effects.

What Others Think About Noni

I am not the only health professional with the opinion that noni can effectively lower high blood pressure. In recent years, noni has been studied at various universities worldwide, including the Stanford University, the University of California at Los Angeles (UCLA), the University of Hawaii, the Union College of London, and at the University of Metz in France.

Another of my colleagues, Scott Gerson, M.D., of the Mt. Sinai School of Medicine in New York, completed a placebo-controlled clinical trial to determine whether noni really could lower high blood pressure. For 14 weeks, Dr. Gerson studied nine hypertensive patients—six males and three females. These patients were selected at random, and did not know that they were taking a noni extract. They stayed on the same diet and maintained the same exercise regimens previous to their beginning the trial. After 14 weeks of noni treatment, eight of the nine patients showed a significant decrease in blood pressure. On average, their systolic pressure (which is the number read on top) dropped by almost 8 percent, and their diastolic pressure (the bottom number) decreased 4 percent.

Dr. Gerson was the first to point out that his clinical trial was not a super-scientific experiment; however, he felt that it did provide solid evidence of noni's ability to lower hypertension and promote a healthier cardiovascular system. His findings were consistent with the results of my survey and of other research. It is important to reiterate that in all the research I have reviewed, of all the doctors I have interviewed, and in all the feedback I have received from thousands of noni users, I have not come across one case where noni lowered blood pressure to below-normal levels. Additionally, reported side effects from those using noni to treat hypertension have been almost nonexistent. It is also interesting to note that many noni users have reported that their high blood pressure returned if they stopped taking noni, then returned again toward normal upon reinstating the noni treatment.

I have received some exciting reports from various doctors who regularly suggest noni as a treatment for high blood pressure. Dr. Mona Harrison, one of today's principal proponents of noni's medicinal value, detailed the account of one of her patients, who had suffered from high blood pressure. Her doctors had been able to lower it to about 170/100, but no more. Turning to Dr. Harrison, she was encouraged to take noni juice. After only two months of taking noni, her blood pressure dropped to a normal, healthier level of 130/80. As of this writing (it has been well over a year), the patient has continued to take noni and has not suffered an increase in blood pressure.

How Noni Helped Me with My Hypertension

"They Ask Me Where To Get the 'Juice!'"

Matthew, from Ontario, Canada, experienced dramatic effects using noni. He explains:

"I have had a number of health problems develop over the last few years. I have a hiatal hernia, high cholesterol levels and high blood pressure. I also suffered a minor stroke in 1994. As one might guess, I have taken numerous medications to treat these conditions.

"I started taking noni juice in March 1997. I was hoping to get my blood pressure under control, so a friend advised me to begin taking two ounces daily—one ounce in the morning and one in the evening. Within the first few days, I noticed that I had more energy and that my hiatal hernia did not "burn" as much as it normally did.

"After another two months or so, my doctor noticed that my blood pressure was normalizing. He asked what I was doing differently, and I told him about the noni. Skeptical, he said that if I wished to continue with the product, that was fine being that it was only a 'fruit juice' and should not hurt me. This continued for another year with the results of my hypertension staying at 120/80. My doctor then asked me if I would supply him with a bottle for himself. This, of course, I did. Soon after, he reported to me that within the first week he also had more energy and an enhanced sense of well-being.

"Within this time, I had mentioned to my doctor that I would like to stop taking my blood pressure medications, especially in light of the success I was having with the noni juice. Hesitant at first, he soon relented to gradually lowering the dosage of my medicines; so we cut my dosage of Adalat XL in half. After about three months on this dose, he agreed that I could quit the Adalat entirely. We will next have testing done to see if I can go off my cholesterol pill.

"I believe that noni has been responsible for the many changes I have recently seen in my health. I believe that because it is a natural product, it can do just as good a job or better than drugs of improving my health, and without side effects. It has given me a new level of energy and overall feeling of improved wellness, all of which has allowed me to get off my medications. As for my doctor, he not only takes noni for himself, but he is also recommending it to other patients (they ask me where to get the "juice"). They, too, are having good results. I will take noni as long as I live!"

"I Don't Dare Stop to Take Noni Juice!"

Raija, from Finland, gives proof that noni can help people from all over the world improve their health. Though her English is somewhat broken, the power of her testimony as to noni's health benefits certainly shines through. She says:

"I have become very inspired by noni juice. I hear about that juice last November and I get interested in it because we in this area of the world have problems with cholesterol in blood and with blood pressure. I also have same problems in my family. Because of problems ordering noni in Finland, I come here [to the U.S.].

"Because I await so long time, when I get that juice I of course drink it many spoonful in one day. I am so ill—head hurt and goes round, my heart hurts. I start with little juice in morning and night. Everybody say to stop to take the juice. Then I take two spoons of juice in the morning and at night. I feeling better and better. I sleep well, I feel well, I don't need hormones or more medications. My heart, my blood pressure getting better. I don't dare stop to take noni juice!"

Raija goes on to note that she has seen similar results in some of her colleagues. For instance, the husband of one of her co-workers also was suffering from high blood pressure and occasional arrhythmias in his heart. On Raija's recommendation, he started taking noni juice, and soon after reported to her that he was able to completely discontinue his hypertension medication and that he had not had a heart arrhythmia since starting on the noni. Raija finishes, "Now he order for his self. . . ."

Complementary Therapies to Noni

As part of a holistic health plan, noni can provide substantial benefits in lowering high blood pressure and improving the health of the heart and cardiovascular system. But there are other areas that can enhance noni's function in fighting hypertension. The following provide other legitimate therapies and treatments for treating high blood pressure and the pursuit of overall improved health.

DIET/NUTRITION RECOMMENDATIONS

Change your diet. Diet is probably the most important factor in both preventing and treating hypertension. Incorporate a diet that is low in high-fat red meat, dairy products, and processed sugar/flour products, and high in whole foods, coldwater fish, and lean white meats. Consume plenty of oat bran, pectin-containing fruits and vegetables, and other fresh fruits and vegetables, including broccoli, cabbage, green leafy vegetables, peas, prunes, beets, and carrots (there are other great options, of course). The incidence of high blood pressure is considerably lower in vegetarians.

Reduce salt intake to moderate levels. Salt encourages the retention of fluid, which contributes to rising blood pressure.

Avoid caffeine. This can temporarily (yet unnecessarily) raise blood pressure.

Increase consumption of garlic and onions. Garlic has been shown to be effective in lowering blood cholesterol levels, as well as in bringing down blood pressure readings. Because many people believe they don't get enough garlic in their diet, they opt for supplementation. Odorless garlic capsules are recommended. Onions provide some of the same benefits as garlic.

Incorporate celery into your diet. Consuming celery, and specifically celery seed and celery oil, have been linked to lowering blood pressure. Celery seed has been used for generations by folk healers and Chinese physicians in the treatment of high blood pressure.

Use more olive and flaxseed oil. If used for cooking and baking purposes, these oils have a health-promoting effect, rather than health-degrading effect. Decrease the use of hydrogenated fats (like margarine).

Eliminate certain foods. Avoid smoked and aged cheeses and meats, chocolate, animal fats, gravies, some canned soups, diet soda, meat tenderizers, soy sauce and ibuprofen medications. These all contain substances, such as monosodium glutamate, that have been linked to high blood pressure and other cardiovascular disease.

SUPPLEMENTATION

Essential fatty acids. Found in fish oils and other plant oils like flaxseed and borage, fatty acids can contribute to the reduction of both high blood pressure and blood lipids. Remember that if taking a fish oil supplement, it is also wise to take a vitamin E supplement.

Vitamin C with bioflavonoids. Studies have shown that supplementing with vitamin C and bioflavonoids may reduce blood pressure.[5] These are compounds that act as free radical scavengers in the arteries and heart muscle.

"Any Drug that Accelerates Your Heart Rate Is Not the Best Solution"

Barry, of Shoreview, Minnesota, relates his incredible experience with noni juice:

"I am a 71-year-old, semi-retired veterinarian, and have been taking noni for about three months. I was told by a friend that it might help stabilize my wildly fluctuating blood pressure. I have been taking different blood pressure medications for at least ten years, and about all I can say is that these drugs will lower your blood pressure, along with your libido, your energy, and your enthusiasm, while at the same time accelerating your heart rate.

"I have been a farmer for 40 years, and I know if you run a machine at a higher speed than it was intended, it will wear out faster. Any drug that accelerates your heart rate to lower blood pressure is not the best solution.

"In addition to my hypertension, I have had other problems. While in vet school, I contracted undulant fever. Though it was diagnosed early, I still suffer from resultant problems, mainly arthritis in my spinal column. Over the years, I have grown increasingly stiff and clumsy, and have lost about three inches off my height. I also suffer from numerous aches, my energy levels have gone downhill, and I have suffered more and more bouts of depression because I could see the end of an active lifestyle. Then I was introduced to noni by a good friend—a nurse—who encouraged me to try noni.

"After a few weeks of taking noni juice, I noticed an improvement in my overall well-being. However, I was disappointed that my blood pressure had not been affected. But my friend wisely counseled me to continue, explaining that just as my condition had taken time to develop, I should then expect it to take some time to reverse itself. So I doubled my dose, making sure to take it on an empty stomach.

"Soon, I really began to notice a real improvement in my energy and enthusiasm. I enjoy using the internet and have often spent two or three hours with my computer in the middle of the night. Even with this sort of interruption in my sleeping, I awaken refreshed and enthused and ready to accomplish my day's activities.

"The other morning, I bicycled six miles to the bank to deposit a check; next door was a drug store with a blood pressure meter. I checked it, and it's as low as it has been in a long, long time— 136/66. That night after supper, my wife needed a few kitchen items, so I hopped on my bike and rode five miles the other way to the store. That means I biked over 20 miles in one day! I was still full of energy and enjoyed my computer until almost midnight. I credit noni juice with giving me a new lease on life!"

Fiber supplement. It is well known that the average American does not get enough dietary fiber, so a fiber supplement can help make up the deficit. Studies show that boosting fiber intake can be a very effective method in treating both high blood pressure and high blood cholesterol levels.[6]

Calcium/magnesium. There is a large body of research linking the deficiency of these two substances to high blood pressure.[7]

Selenium. Deficiencies of this mineral have also been linked to high blood pressure and heart disease. Because most diets are lacking in this mineral, supplementation may be vital.[8]

Herbal combination containing cayenne, chamomile, fennel, hawthorn berries and rosemary. These and other herbs have been used for centuries to treat the various symptoms of heart disease.

Valerian, hops and kava. These three herbs can help relieve anxiety, which can play a role in high blood pressure.

Coenzyme Q10. This valuable substance has been shown to possess multiple health benefits, among them improving the health of the heart and related tissues. It has also been shown to help lower hypertension.[9]

OTHER RECOMMENDATIONS

Don't smoke. As we discussed earlier in the chapter, smoking is one of the "big three" factors for increasing the risk of stroke and heart attack. It also goes without saying that not smoking produces a number of other health benefits as well.

Get rid of excess weight. Another of the "big three" risk factors for stroke and heart attack, being overweight can be dealt with through various factors, diet and exercise being the most effective. There are numerous studies proving that excess weight dramatically increases one's risk of developing hypertension and other related cardiovascular conditions, and premature death.

Implement a stress-reduction program. An impressive body of research reveals that relieving stress can significantly reduce high blood pressure levels. Meditation techniques can diffuse stress, leading to lower blood pressure. Other therapies, such as relaxation techniques and exercise, can significantly reduce mental and emotional stress, which can ultimately lead to a more normal blood pressure.

Exercise. This one is simple: exercising for at least a half hour, three times weekly, can do wonders for high blood pressure. It has numerous other benefits as well.

Have your blood pressure checked regularly. This can be done either at home or by your doctor, and will help you track your progress in improving your condition.

Chapter Summary Points

• High blood pressure, one of today's most prevalent health conditions in the U.S. and other Western countries, is really just an indicator of an underlying problem in the cardiovascular system.
• Because high blood pressure can be largely controlled through special attention on diet, exercise and other factors, noni can help lower

high blood pressure towards normal levels if incorporated into a holistic health plan.

• There is considerable research indicating that noni either contains or stimulates the production of a number of substances than can help lower high blood pressure. Most notable among these are scopoletin and nitric oxide, both of which are proven antihypertension agents.

• My survey of noni users and other health professionals using noni found that an overwhelming number of those using noni to treat their hypertension experienced a measurable lowering of their high blood pressure and related problems.

Noni and Chronic Pain

DON RECOUNTS HIS harrowing experience from a climbing accident and his subsequent recovery using noni juice:

"In the fall of 1996, I was on what I thought was going to be a regular Boy Scout camping trip. After camping Friday night, we woke the next morning and climbed to the top of a two-hundred-foot cliff. I could never have imagined what would happen to me in the following hours, days and months.

"As I began my usual review with the boys on the ins and outs of rappelling, we tied off ropes, pulled on gloves and tightened our harnesses. After these preparations, I hooked into the rope in the usual manner and began climbing over the edge. Once I was over the edge and the rope was laying on the rock, I knew it was safe to jump out and down the rocky terrain. I was only about 10–15 feet over the edge of a cliff that was about 200 feet high when I looked up to see the rope sliding across the rock at the top and cut completely apart. I gasped as my breath left me and pushed off the rock face as hard as I could. I was trying to push off to the other side, as I was over a ravine, and land on the face of the other cliff. But I was not able to, and I instead hit and bounced back and forth until I landed in a crevice and slid about 20 feet where I finally came to a stop. Not surprisingly, I blacked out for a time.

"When I came to, I opened my eyes and looked into the face of a friend and asked, "Am I going to die?" I was able, through a rush of adrenaline, to move myself up to the top of the cliff, where I collapsed and laid there in agony until a rescue team arrived. After a bumpy ride in a truck and helicopter, I at last arrived at a hospital.

"My injuries were serious and varied. My left elbow had a severe cut; I had broken both wrists and a finger; my jaw was broken in two places near the joint at the ears and shattered in front; the lower jaw was dislocated, pushing up into the skull; my right cheek bone was broken and had to be wired back together; finally, my right nasal passage was damaged, but I felt lucky to be alive!

"My recovery was painful and difficult. I spent six days in the hospital, then had my mouth wired shut for six weeks, wearing wires and steel bars with heavy-duty rubber bands on my mouth for another three weeks. I spent two months in a wheel chair and another several weeks on crutches. I also had to have surgery to help my bones repair themselves correctly.

"About six weeks into my recovery, a friend called and told me of a product—Tahitian Noni Juice™—that might be able to help. Of course, I told him about the extreme difficulty I was having moving around, rising from a sitting position, and the persistent and sometimes unbearable pain all over my body. I also was extremely tired, taking naps constantly without ever recovering much of my strength or energy. What could possibly help me?

"But I agreed to take noni juice, and decided to drop all my other medications to see if noni really helped. I didn't notice any real changes for the first few days, but on the fifth morning, I noticed a very distinct change. I got right out of bed and raised myself right up! I couldn't quite believe that it was the noni, but I kept taking it, increasing the dosage to five total ounces per day.

"The results I experienced after that were incredible. I was immediately able to stay up all day and sit at the computer and work. I was able to type, one finger at a time, and noticed a big increase in energy every day. After about a week, I was "popping" out of bed every morning at 7 a.m. (with no alarm clock), not needing a nap all day and working until midnight. And, the pain I was previously experiencing was minimal and irregular.

"Shortly after this time, I had all the remaining wires, bars and rubber bands taken off my mouth, but during the process of positioning my chin, the doctor noticed the front of the chin was not closed up. This would probably result in my getting a bone graft to close the opening. His instructions were to stick with the liquid diet I was on, and in one month we would re-examine it to determine if I would need the bone graft. I stuck with the noni juice, and after the month had passed and the doctor examined my chin, we were both surprised and pleased to find that the opening was healing properly; consequently, I would not need the bone graft.

"To say the least, I was elated! I firmly believe that noni played a primary role in my speedy and efficient recovery, my increase in energy levels and the reduction of the pain and soreness that I was suffering from. I would advise anyone who might be hesitant to take the product—it is entirely worth it. I thank God for bringing this product to me in my time of need!"

Not everyone is as fortunate as Don. Many people experience the debilitating shift from acute pain to chronic pain. If you are one of those people, you probably feel frightened and alone. You may feel helpless. You might even feel as if life is no longer worth living. Being in pain, hour after hour, day after day, rips away your strength, your personality, your hope, and even your love. You have one of the worst medical problems a person can have. Physically devastating, chronic pain can be even more overwhelming than having a terminal illness, according to sufferers of both conditions.

This is what happened to Cory. A middle-aged man, he looked much older—his skin was a pale, milky color, though his face was bloated and acne pocked from the steroids and anti-inflammatory drugs he was taking. He was very thin, though at a younger age he weighed a healthy 185 pounds. And he was angry—angry at the drugs, angry at his pain, angry at his doctor, but most of all, angry at life itself. But who could blame him? His life was one of constant, severe and widespread pain.

Cory suffered from lupus erythematosus, an autoimmune disease that manifests itself in many ways, and is a disease that science has yet to comprehensively grasp what it really is. For many sufferers, lupus is more of an inconvenience than a full-blown disease. But for others, including people like Cory, lupus can be an excruciating, entirely engulfing state of hell. After years of various treatments involving all kinds of drugs, numerous hospitalizations, constant fatigue, an almost

The Modern Epidemic of Chronic Pain

Why It's Occurring

- More people than ever before are older than forty-five, the "magic age" for vulnerability to chronic pain.
- More people are surviving degenerative diseases, such as cancer. However, despite surviving the condition, they are more prone to its debilitating effects, such as pain.
- More people are surviving accidents. Like the previous bullet explains, higher survival rates mean higher rates of suffering after the accident.
- More people than ever maintain extremely high stress levels.
- More people than ever are sedentary (meaning they don't exercise) and overweight.

How Widespread is the Epidemic?

- Chronic pain causes more disability than heart disease and cancer combined.
- More than a quarter of all Americans experience some form of chronic pain each year, including arthritis and back pain.
- About 13 percent of Americans—or 20 million people—experience chronic pain on half of all the days in a year.
- Pain is one of the top three reasons for visiting the doctor.
- Nearly 15 percent of American women suffer from migraine headaches.

complete loss of social life, and episodes of deep depression, Cory had been told that his pain was essentially inescapable.

Chronic pain can result from various sources. And like many health conditions, there are many levels of pain a sufferer may experience. But what is chronic pain? Despite being such a common complaint, many doctors don't really understand what chronic pain is. Some think that chronic pain is basically the same as short-term "acute" pain. They believe that chronic pain is just acute pain that lasts longer.

That's not true. As we'll examine more closely, chronic pain, though maybe originally a symptom of an underlying condition, usually ends up becoming its own condition, its own disease. But chronic pain can be treated, and some doctors have developed rigorous and effective holistic health regimens to relieve pain. When incorporated into a holistic health plan, the exciting food supplement noni has been shown to help those suffering from chronic pain not only get rid of the pain, but regain the satisfying aspects of their life as well.

How Pain Works

For years, scientists and doctors have not had a complete enough understanding of pain; therefore, pain treatments have usually been centered around drugs that partially or temporarily cut off pain without healing its underlying cause. One need only look at the plethora of over-the-counter and prescription drugs designed strictly to mask pain. If there were one that completely rid the body of pain over the long-term, there would not be so many medications fighting for your dollars.

However, recent research and investigative data in the area of pain and chronic illness has revealed that chronic pain can indeed be reversed through holistic and "natural" means, to allow for a more normal and rewarding life. These treatments have come about because of a fundamental understanding of what pain really is and how it really works.

According to Dr. Dharma Singh Khalsa, author of *The Pain Cure,* pain works within its own nervous system pathway that contains biological "gates" that can be closed to shut off pain. When these gates are closed, the pain is reduced or even eliminated. This concept is often referred to as the "gate theory," and it has brought a much more in-depth understanding that has revolutionized the world of pain management.[1]

This theory, now increasingly being incorporated into the treatment programs of many pain specialists, is still relatively new. Therefore, many doctors not specializing in pain management may not be aware of how this fits into their regimens. Because of this, and as many sufferers of chronic pain know, modern medical treatments may be incomplete. In fact, as I mentioned earlier, many doctors don't really understand what chronic pain is, often mistaking it for long-term "acute" pain instead of a chronic malfunction of the nervous system.

This point brings us to the question of how pain works. A painful impulse usually begins its trip along the pain pathway when you suffer an injury or illness—say, a broken bone. These impulses pass through various "gates" along the way, and will end up at one point in the brain, which then processes and sends the impulse back to the injured area, sensitizing the area and causing inflammation or other localized changes. The sensitizing and inflammation help to protect the damaged area by forcing us to favor it and rushing healing biochemicals to the area. However, sensitizing and inflammation can magnify the pain or even create new pain. This new pain travels back to the brain via the various biological gates—and the cycle once again begins.

As the pain signals come and go, come and go, it is easy to see how the cycle can become "engraved" upon the nervous system pathways, causing various elements of chronic pain syndrome to "jam" open the gates of the pain pathway and to magnify the sensations of pain. Eventually these sensations, traveling back and forth and causing more pain, can effectively take on a life of their own. At this point, it is not just a symptom or result of the injury. Instead, it has become its own entity, its own disease. It has become chronic pain.

Defending Against Pain

The body employs a number of ways to fight pain and its debilitating effects. Let's say that you cut your arm. You have probably noticed that when you cut or injure yourself, you typically feel the sensation of being cut before you actually feel any pain from the cut. That is because you have separate nerves for touch, pain and other sensations, and the "touch" nerves are able to send their signals much more quickly than those nerves that send pain signals. So, that's why you usually "sense" the cut before you feel pain from it.

After you cut your arm, you automatically reach for it to squeeze and rub it, right? That natural instinct surfaces because it decreases your pain. Why? Because rubbing or squeezing the injured area sends faster "touch" signals, which outrun the slower "pain" signals. By the time the pain signals arrive at their respective receptor sites, the touch impulses have crowded them, leaving little space for the pain signals to squeeze through. This is one simple way to fight pain—to send a natural response of rubbing, squeezing and touching the injured area that compete against and outrun pain impulses.

There are other ways the body battles pain. When pain signals begin their journey to the brain, they automatically trigger a release of several chemicals that can flood the brain, giving physical and physiological relief. These substances, referred to as "opiates," not only provide relief from pain signals in the brain, they also travel to one of the pain "gates" in the spine, where they battle the pain-carrying substance-P, trying to keep it from entering the nerves that go to the brain. Some of the more important opiates include endorphins, dynorphins, and enkephalins, all of which provide strength ten times that of morphine. Fortunately, the human body never builds up tolerance to them as it does to morphine and other drugs.

There is one more way the body can battle pain. That is through the adequate production and utilization of serotonin, a valuable biochemical that helps maintain the proper elasticity in blood vessels, which

Common Side Effects of Pain Drugs

(The most common drugs include sedatives, NSAIDs, analgesics, beta-blockers, antidepressants, and muscle relaxers)

- memory loss
- depression
- kidney damage
- stroke
- lethargy
- heart disease
- osteoporosis

- anxiety
- liver damage
- high blood pressure
- insomnia
- vomiting/nausea
- rashes
- ulcers

helps prevent pain common to such ailments as migraine headaches. I'll talk a bit more about serotonin—and its relationship with noni—later in this chapter.

How the Healing Process Can Hurt

Let's talk briefly about another problem pain sufferers may face. Generally, in response to minor injuries, the body plays it safe, organizing a "defensive" protection against the injury until it is certain that all is well. However, when the body (and specifically the brain) realize that the pain signals it is receiving are severe in nature, it launches a counterattack. While this reaction needs to be strong to control the onslaught of pain signals, if it is too strong it can lead to more long-lasting problems like chronic pain. For instance, instead of telling your neurotransmitter system to pump out calming neurotransmitters, your brain puts in an order for the stimulating neurotransmitter norepinephrine, a form of adrenaline. This usually happens when your body is under assault, and suddenly, you begin to experience the classic symptoms of the "fight-or-flight" response. Your blood vessels constrict, your heart pounds, your muscles tighten and your nerves go "on edge" as your body waits for other problems.

This can be the first step down the path to chronic pain. If your body is continually involved in the production of stimulants, instead of maintaining a balance of stimulants and relaxants, then the gates through which pain impulses pass can, and will, eventually become "jammed" open.

Compound this with another problem. The natural opiates, like norepinephrine, that your body creates, can run out. If you don't have enough, then the pain signals have one less obstacle to overcome. When this happens, the signals, if frequent and intense enough, can themselves jam open the pain gates, leaving the path free to travel to and from the brain without obstruction. As this happens—millions of times per hour—pain signals can literally become engraved upon the nervous system. Thus the pain signals become a physical part of the

The Biological Pain "Gateways"
(taken from The Pain Cure, by Dharma Singh Khalsa, M.D.)

What opens them (and increases pain)	**What closes them** (and decreases pain)
• lack of sleep	• relaxation
• fear/anxiety about pain	• exercise
• stressful lifestyle	• medications
• depression	• adequate serotonin levels
• repeated injury	• acupuncture
• physical inactivity	• physical activity
• lack of specific nutrients	• abundance of nutrients
• obsession with pain	• distraction from pain
• endorphin deficit	• normal level of endorphins
• hypoglycemia	• meditation
• serotonin deficit	• mental training

anatomy of your nervous system, no matter that the original injury has healed.

Like we've seen earlier, when this occurs the pain is no longer a symptom. Instead, it has become its own health condition. It has become chronic pain.

Relieving the Pain: Noni's Analgesic Effects

This brings our discussion to noni and how it can help fight chronic pain. A review of the historical literature concerning noni's health benefits reveals that one of its most popular uses in folk medicine was to relieve most types of pain, be it chronic or acute. From the Eastern medicine healers of Southeast Asia to the Hawaiian kahunas to Caribbean folk doctors, the notion that noni could (and can) effectively treat pain is quite apparent.

But what about noni's modern uses? A short time after beginning my investigation into noni and its effects on human health, I soon realized that one of the more common ailments for which people are now using noni is chronic pain, whether from arthritis, headaches, or other chronic conditions. It was no surprise, then, when I discovered that this was also the case with the various doctors from whom I was receiving correspondence. Case after case and history after history showed that taking noni juice can produce both dramatic and gradual results in conditions from severe arthritic pain to dull, nagging back pain to occasional migraine headaches.

One such doctor, Mona Harrison, M.D., has continually studied the latest in food supplements and alternative health therapies to provide her patients with the best care possible. After learning about noni in 1997 from one of her staff members (who, after only two weeks of taking noni, noticed a terrific improvement in her varicose veins and a chronic digestive ailment), Dr. Harrison decided that she would give noni a try.

Consequently, she sent a package containing noni and some literature to several of her patients, explaining that she wanted to get firsthand feedback on noni if they were willing to try the juice.

The results were spectacular. She received reports back from cancer patients, individuals with severe vision problems, and liver disease. But one of the more incredible accounts involved a woman who had been suffering from degenerative arthritis for more than 20 years. Because the arthritis was so bad, both her knees had to be replaced. Despite this drastic measure, however, there was little alleviation in her pain. The woman still had to walk with a cane, and had a terrible time rising from a sitting position.

After using Dr. Harrison's noni for just 72 hours, this patient enthusiastically reported to Dr. Harrison that she could get up from a soft-cushioned sofa and walk across the room without a cane—or pain, for that matter. She was certain that it was the noni that produced such a dramatic result because it was the only variable that had changed in her life.

Another medical professional, Dr. Delbert Hatton, a chiropractic physician, recalls his personal experience with noni and chronic pain. For approximately forty years, Dr. Hatton has suffered from a constant, nagging ache in his lower back from unevenly formed vertebrae.

The pain prevented him from doing many of the things he enjoys, and didn't even let him participate in normal household and yard-keeping duties. After only six weeks of taking noni, his back pain disappeared. He says that after starting to recommend noni to his patients about two years ago, he has had remarkable success in most cases.

One example of success with Dr. Hatton's patients involved a man injured in a traumatic auto accident. He broke several ribs, his shoulder and his knee. Because of these injuries, he developed severe arthritis in several areas of his body, but especially his knee. Only days after he started taking noni juice, the patient experienced a dramatic lessening of pain in his knee and a more gradual decrease of pain in his ribs and shoulder. Currently, he is virtually pain-free.

Dr. Hatton provides still another success story involving noni and the treatment of pain. This particular patient broke several bones in her ankle, and consequently suffered from lingering pain and swelling in the area for more than a year and a half. A mere ten days after starting to take noni, the woman reported that both the pain and swelling decreased substantially. Dr. Hatton attributes this to noni's ability to enhance the individual cells' ability to assimilate and utilize the needed nutrients to facilitate repair of diseased or damaged cells and tissue. Dr. Hatton is so enthusiastic about noni's varied health benefits that he declared to me that he would feel confident about noni's chances of successfully treating any kind of health problem.

Another doctor whose experience with noni has been quite impressive is Dr. Gary Tran, a veterinarian who has treated more than 5,000 animals with noni. Dr. Tran first heard about noni nearly three years ago, but he was somewhat skeptical of its abilities. But he finally convinced himself to try it. That very day, his aunt called to tell him that her daughter was dying of AIDS. So he sent a case of noni juice to his cousin, explaining its reported health benefits. Not long after, his cousin reported to him that noni had helped her immensely. So he decided to use it for himself, as well as to give it to his family. It helped with his wife's chronic fatigue syndrome and his son's debilitating migraine headaches. And Dr. Tran even received personal benefit from the noni—short-term treatment eased his own arthritis and asthma.

Both intrigued and convinced by these results, Dr. Tran decided to bring this seemingly miracle fruit to his four-legged patients. He reports that noni has helped more than 90 percent of the animals to which he has given noni, noting that "noni is not only wonderful for alleviating pain, but it's also antihistaminic, anthelmintic (rids animals of worms), anti-inflammatory, analgesic, and anticarcinogenic."[2] He adds that he has used noni to treat an enormous variety of conditions for his animal patients, including neurological disorders, spinal cord injuries, sprains, fractures, arthritis, joint problems, inflammation, and more. Most convincing is the fact that Dr. Tran no longer has so much need of traditional pain-killing drugs, muscle relaxants or steroids in the majority of his animal clients. Instead he uses noni juice.

Pain Relief: How Noni Does It

As I mentioned earlier, noni is evidently a potent pain-relief agent. Literally thousands of current users, as well as a large body of historical materials, attest to this notion. But this leads one to ask exactly how noni relieves pain. The fact is, there is no clear answer. However, with the available scientific research into other areas of noni, coupled with the abundance of specific and detailed clinical use, there exist several plausible theories as to how noni can provide definite and even dramatic relief for chronic pain sufferers. Some believe that the xeronine system is solely responsible for noni's pain relief abilities. Others think that noni's ability to enhance the utilization of necessary nutrients in "sick" cells may be the answer. Paul Cox, one of the world's top ethnobotanists, confirmed to me in personal conversations what I had learned from several kahunas concerning their pain treatment secrets: that the spiritual magic of noni comes from "pule" (prayer) and originates "from within."[3] In other words, despite the fact that the theories surrounding noni's antipain benefits are varied, noni's ability to fight pain is certainly evident.

Science may have a little more to say about noni's health benefits. In 1992, Julia Morton, a noted botanist, reported that noni contains ter-

• back pain	• angina
• chronic fatigue syndrome	• cancer
• osteoarthritis	• rheumatoid arthritis
• bursitis	• tendinitis
• fractures	• wounds
• injury recovery	• migraines
• headaches (general)	• lupus
• dental work/toothache	• fibromyalgia
• stress headaches	• sinusitis
• ulcers	• Crohn's disease
• diverticulitis	• irritable bowel syndrome
• reproductive system disorders	• carpal tunnel syndrome

Table 8.1: **Sources of chronic pain against which noni may be effective (taken from findings of scientific research, informal surveys, and testimonial material).**

penes, found in essential oils, that have been shown to aid in cell synthesis and cell rejuvenation. Other recent research reveals that noni contains numerous known essential nutrients, including proteins, amino acids, enzymes, vitamins and minerals, that may synergistically contribute to noni's ability to fight pain and a host of other ailments. Richard Dicks, a New Jersey naturopathic educator, cites his personal experience with noni, giving an explanation similar to this. His son had severe bone disease and arthritis, experiencing severe pain from a very young age. When Richard heard about noni from a friend, he decided to do his own detective work. For eight months, he took noni himself and gave it to his son without telling anyone. Richard told me in an interview that noni was his "secret agent."

The results were astounding. Richard's son's pain dissipated to the point that it was almost entirely gone. How did this happen? Richard attributes the results to noni's effectiveness in cell regeneration and the provision of vital nutrients that help the body battle any condition, whether it be chronic pain or an ear infection. Says Richard, "We're beginning to realize that we must get back to basics with our bodies. What it boils down to is either burn nutrients or burn your body. Noni saves our bodies by giving us the nutrients we need."[4]

Serotonin and the Xeronine System

I believe that noni does provide a number of necessary compounds, biochemicals and other nutrients that allow our cells to regenerate quickly and properly, and thereby facilitating the reversal of a wide variety of health conditions, including pain. Remember our earlier discussion of xeronine and the Golgi apparatus? We examined how xeronine (formed from proxeronine and proxeroninase) works hand in hand with the nerve cells' Golgi apparatus to package and deliver necessary bundles of nutrients to damaged, sick and malfunctioning cells. After reviewing the literature available on noni, and having extensive correspondence and conversations with Dr. Ralph Heinicke and others, I believe that one of these nutrients whose capabilities are enhanced by the presence of xeronine is serotonin, a neurotransmitter with a full armory of health benefits.

Recent years have expanded our knowledge of serotonin and the multiple roles it plays in relieving conditions like depression, anxiety, and sleep dysfunction. It achieves these things largely because of the role it plays in the brain and nervous system. Dr. Heinicke's extensive research revealing noni's part in the body's production and proper utilization of serotonin provides us with exciting possibilities as to how noni relieves pain. We know that serotonin, triggered by the brain, tells the nerves that first pick up the pain signal to "calm down," causing the muscles and blood vessels around the injured areas to relax. Your body loosens up, causing the pain to subside and letting you get back to feeling fine.

UNDERSTANDING CHRONIC MIGRAINE PAIN

We also know that because of serotonin's ability to relax constricted blood vessels, it can help alleviate the pain of chronic migraines. As many migraine sufferers know, their headaches begin when blood vessels in the brain suddenly expand and contract, which encourages them to slowly leak blood, which ultimately leads to irritated nerves in the skull lining. So, in a sense, migraines are a form of inflammation.[5]

But what makes the blood vessels in the brain expand and constrict? Often, the cause is eating foods that contain the amino acid tyramine. These include wine, aged cheese, and caffeine. Of course, stress can also be a culprit. There are other reports that link things like carbon monoxide and perfume to blood vessel constriction.

However, most people exposed to these things do not get migraines. This is because they have plenty of the substance needed to properly regulate the constriction and relaxation of blood vessels. And not only does this chemical stop constriction, but it also allows blood vessels to constrict temporarily without quickly expanding. This chemical, of course, is serotonin.

Dr. Khalsa believes that serotonin levels are one of the key indicators in determining migraine severity and frequency. He provides the following reasons:

- One of today's most effective migraine drugs, sumatriptan, works by mimicking the effects of serotonin.
- Almost all migraine patients have limited ability to retain serotonin in their blood platelet membranes.
- Migraines are almost always preceded by a decline in blood levels of serotonin.
- As a rule, low levels of serotonin in the blood accurately predict vulnerability to migraines.
- Disruption of estrogen levels—which markedly decreases serotonin—is a prime trigger of migraines.

Dr. Khalsa goes on to state that normalizing serotonin levels in the body can help alleviate the effects of migraines by more ways than just improving the elasticity of blood vessels. These include raising the brain's pain threshold, promoting healthy sleep patterns, reducing pain-amplifying anxiety, and reducing pain-amplifying depression.[6]

THE LINK BETWEEN NONI AND SEROTONIN

So what's the connection between noni and serotonin? While there is no direct proof, research carried out by Dr. Heinicke and others

"Medically Unprecedented"

Dr. Russel Cooper, a holistic medical practitioner from Australia, gives a powerful account of noni's impressive ability to relieve pain:

"For 26 years, I have had active ankylosing spondylitis, an autoimmune disease that causes extensive and relentless inflammation, stiffness, rigidity, and ultimately the fusing of the spine, hips, neck and random peripheral joints like the knees, ankles, shoulders and fingers. At times, my pain would be so severe that I would not be able to roll over in bed at night due to total back and neck spasms and intense pain.

"I started non-steroidal anti-inflammatory drugs (NSAIDs) and have taken them every single day for the last 18 years. I would experience severe pain when the tablets' effect wore off, then would use meditation, hot baths, and cold showers to manage. With my training in nutritional medicine, I was able to reduce the dose of the NSAIDs by using natural anti-inflammatory preparations, but I was never able to completely stop.

"Just about a year ago, I was introduced to noni juice. Within three days of taking it, I noticed less pain and stiffness. After one week, I did not take my anti-inflammatory tablet for one night, and did not have any 'rebound' stiffness the next day. After two weeks of taking noni, I stopped taking the NSAID tablet for two nights and again had no 'rebound' stiffness. After three weeks on noni, I stopped taking my NSAID tablets completely, and have not taken one since.

"What is more amazing is that I have regained movement in my neck and back, which is virtually medically unprecedented. I have gained vertical height, lost weight and gained muscle since beginning my noni treatment. I can say with a certainty that noni has been transformational in my life!"

Dr. Cooper relates another incredible experience that attests to noni's pain-fighting capabilities:

"Just a few months ago, my half-ton truck rolled off a bank on my bush property and my legs were trapped above the ankles underneath the truck. No one was around. I was able to use my cellular phone to call neighbors and the ambulance. By the time the ambulance arrived, I had lost feeling in my feet and my circulation was threatened. I was in physiological shock. Forty minutes after the accident, the truck was hydraulically airlifted off my legs. Immediately, I drank half a bottle of noni juice and the other half in the next few hours. I also applied noni directly to the puncture wounds and used a noni compress over the crushed tissue.

"How well did the noni work? Amazingly, I had absolutely not a single bruise on either leg nor any neuralgia (nerve pain) following the accident. In addition, the next day I worked in my medical practice from nine in the morning to six that evening. During the course of my recovery, I did not need to take a single conventional analgesic, and the wounds never became infected and healed swiftly without the need of antibiotics.

"Needless to say, I know of no other substance—natural or conventional—that could have produced this extraordinary result. Noni juice truly is amazing."

suggests that noni works with serotonin in the body to alleviate a number of conditions, including pain resulting from arthritis, autoimmune disorders and migraines. In chapter 4, I discuss how the body uses an efficient, yet little-known, portion of the body's cells to package and send bundles of nutrients to needy cells. This area of the cell is called the Golgi apparatus. I believe, as does Dr. Heinicke (often referred to as the Heinicke-Solomon theory) that xeronine plays a central role in helping the Golgi apparatus achieve the proper "packaging" and "shipping" of these nutrient bundles to damaged cells.

Moreover, there is the strong possibility that in these bundles of nutrients will be found pain-fighting substances like serotonin. As we have already shown, the body uses serotonin to fight pain in a number of ways. But the body can't take advantage of the serotonin if it isn't present within the suffering area. I suspect that one way serotonin becomes available for an affected area is through a smooth-functioning Golgi apparatus that, through the help of the xeronine system, safely and efficiently delivers the serotonin package to the intended target.

How Noni Helped Me Get Rid of the Pain

"My Husband Has Never Seen Me Like This!"

Beatrice S. explains how noni helped her reverse her chronic pain, inflammation and depression:

"As a young girl, I contracted polio. Though lucky to survive, I was told that as I grew older, I would probably develop severe arthritis. They were right—I began to suffer from it almost immediately after. From there, it just got worse.

"I had several doctors—all of them gave me all kinds of drugs, old and new. Some worked for a few weeks, but then my body just seemed to grow numb to their effects. Soon, all the steroids and drugs did was make me gain weight and become very depressed.

"Now, forty years later, I had my left knee replaced (it became extremely stiff and never worked right), and my rheumatologist has told me that because of the severity of my pain, the best thing to do is have all my joints—ankles, knees, hips, wrists and shoulders— replaced. He suggested that I have my spine and neck fused as well. That was very discouraging.

"Things at home were terrible. The pain was so unbearable that I had to have my eleven-year-old bathe and dress me. When my husband arrived home from work, he would have to turn me every 20 minutes or so. My son would offer to help me or get something for me, and I would yell at him to leave me alone. Once he turned at the door and said, 'Mom, I know you love me and don't mean a word you said— it's just because you're hurting so much that made you say them. It's okay, I understand that.' Needless to say, I cried all the more.

"In January 1996, I was planning on committing suicide, and told my parents so. My father told me to just fight for a little longer. A couple of days later, a friend of mine told me about a product that could probably help me. When she came over with a bottle of noni juice, I laughed at her, asking what fruit juice would do for me. But I consented to try it, seeing that it certainly couldn't hurt me.

"So, I took two tablespoons that afternoon and two more before going to bed. The next day, I noticed that I wasn't as tired, and my pain, though still present, wasn't as sharp. I told my husband what I had noticed: he said he thought I was a bit more at ease. Before going to sleep that night, I prayed that this juice be the miracle I was looking for.

"That night, I nearly scared my husband to death. When he woke up to turn me, instead of facing away from him, as he had positioned me before going to sleep, I was now facing him. I had not turned by myself in a very long time. That morning, I decided to try and get out of bed by myself for the first time in years. My husband wasn't so keen on the idea, but he stood by and watched as I did it. We were so happy! That was a good day. Though it was only the second day I had taken noni, my pain was not nearly so persistent and severe.

"That evening, I told Rick (my husband) not to worry about waking to turn me. In the morning, I had turned myself, just like the previous night. As Rick was helping our son get ready for school, I decided to get up on my own again to go to the bathroom. Without realizing it, I walked down the hall without my canes. I became nervous, and reached out and grabbed the closet door. I thought I could hold on to the walls and furniture to get into the living room where my walker was. I thought to myself, 'I've come this far—why not go on?' As I passed into the living room, both my son and husband came in. I will never forget the look on their faces. Anthony stood there yelling, 'Mom, you're walking! You're walking!' Rick asked me if I realized what I was doing. I cried and laughed a happy 'yes.' That night, I went to my boy's room to tuck him in. I heard him talking, so I moved in quietly. He was praying to God, thanking him for noni juice and my friend that brought it over. He then asked God to lead him down the roads that had empty cans so he could sell them to get enough money to buy the noni juice for me. I bumped his door, and he quickly turned to me, tears running down his face.

"'What's wrong?' I asked. He said, 'Mom, I am eleven years old, and this is the first time I remember you tucking me into bed.' We had lots of tears that night. All this on only the third day of using noni. Since that day, I have not used my crutches, canes, walker, or wheelchair. They're all up in the attic, collecting dust.

"The amazing results did not stop there. My pain and stiffness had diminished so much that I was able to clean my friend's house two weeks later. We also drove to another town, where I danced with both my husband and my son. The next day, I enjoyed a fantastic day of swimming and going down water slides.

"I am so happy my daddy asked me to fight just a little longer, and that my friend brought the miraculous blessing of noni into our lives. I feel like I need to tell everyone I see about how noni can make them healthy. I thought my life was over, but thanks to noni, it has just begun. I used to beg God to give me just five minutes free of pain. Now I enjoy normal life. My husband has never seen me like this. Needless to say, I thank God every morning and evening.

"About a year ago, I went to the doctor. She had not seen me since I was able to walk on my own. She was completely shocked and wanted to know what happened. I was more than happy to tell her about noni. So she did an x-ray of my knee, and determined that the entire knee was not so deformed and was recovering its normal structure. She didn't know what to say, other than that I was obviously not in pain and to come back when I got sick. Well, with noni juice, I'm not planning on any doctor visits soon."

Complementary Therapies to Noni

Despite the overwhelming evidence that noni can promote pain relief on its own, there are a number of things you can do to further noni's effectiveness and complement its abilities.

DIETARY/SUPPLEMENTATION CONSIDERATIONS

Increasing the level of the following nutrients in one's diet, or supplementing with these supplements can provide additional firepower in fighting pain:

EPA (eicosapentaenoic acid). A fatty acid that comes from fish such as salmon, tuna, and mackerel, this fatty acid can help normalize the body's inflammation response. It can be effective against inflammatory diseases such as rheumatoid arthritis.

GLA (gamma linolenic acid). This fat is similar to EPA, though its benefits don't seem to be quite as strong as those of EPA. It can be taken in supplement form, usually sold as evening primrose oil. It could be helpful used in combinations with other fatty acids.

ALA (alpha linolenic acid). Found mostly in green vegetables, this is not usually found in supplement form. Great sources of ALA include the chlorophyll-filled "green foods" such as spirulina, wheat grass, alfalfa and chlorella. These foods also contain a number of other very important nutrients, all of which can contribute to the reduction of inflammation and pain.

Turmeric. A spice commonly used in Eastern food dishes, turmeric contains high levels of curcumin, a substance often shown to be as effective as anti-inflammatories like cortisone, ibuprofen and phenylbutazone. Unlike these drugs, however, curcumin is very safe, even when taken in high doses. Studies have shown turmeric (and specifically curcumin) to be effective against rheumatoid arthritis and general joint stiffness and swelling.

Chamomile. This pleasant-tasting herb is an effective anti-inflammatory agent, as well as a mild sedative. It also helps relieve muscle spasms. It has been shown to specifically help with trigeminal neuralgia (facial nerve pain). Chamomile can be used in teas, capsules or compresses.

Cayenne. Also known as capsicum, this red chile pepper provides "warmth" that gives a stimulant to the brain that competes with pain signals. It has been shown to prevent the production of substance-P, a pain-carrying chemical.

DL-phenylalanine. This amino acid form helps fight pain, preventing the breakdown of endorphins. Studies have shown it to be especially effective against chronic pain.[7]

White willow bark. A very popular herbal, white willow contains salicin, which is converted to salicylic acid, similar to aspirin. It has been used for centuries in various cultures for treating numerous types of aches and pains.

Phosphatidyl serine. This substance aids the nerve cells in conducting impulses, helps the brain to manufacture neurotransmitters and blocks the stress hormone cortisol, which can contribute to an increased perception of pain. It has been shown in a number of studies to improve short-term memory and concentration, which are important in the body's control of pain.

Avoid animal fats. Animal meats, like red meat, pork, and chicken contain fats and other substances that can contribute to symptoms of arthritis, inflammation and general joint pain.

OTHER CONSIDERATIONS

As the chapter explains, pain is a complex entity that can accompany other disorders or become its own condition. Because of this, there are a substantial number of treatments or therapies—and too many, frankly, to discuss here—that may help alleviate pain. My suggestion would be to consult one or more of the many excellent reference texts available that adequately outline commonly used and effective antipain therapies. Consulting health care providers familiar with these therapies can also be very helpful. With my patients, I found the following antipain therapies to be helpful: hypnosis, imagery, total muscle relaxation, abdominal breathing, visualization, distraction, focusing, and mental anesthesia.

Chapter Summary Points

- Chronic pain can result from an underlying ailment (such as arthritis or an injury) and eventually become its own condition.
- Many pain experts believe that pain travels along its own nervous system pathways, which contain gates that open and close. If the gates are closed, the pain can't travel and therefore is minimized. It is believed by many that these gates can begin to malfunction and become "jammed," which allows pain signals to travel continuously and therefore contribute to a condition of chronic pain.
- Chronic pain is one of the most common complaints for which noni has been utilized, both historically and in modern times. Because pain is associated with such a wide variety of ailments, it is one of the most oft-reported symptoms alleviated by noni use.
- Though it is not completely clear how noni works so effectively as an antipain agent, it is clear that most people using it to help relieve their pain find it to be very powerful. My survey of noni users and health professionals who use noni in their work found that 87 percent of the more than 3,700 people taking it for pain were successful in alleviating the pain with noni. And those taking it for ailments highly associated with pain, such as arthritis, experienced similar results.
- I believe, as do other health experts, that noni's antipain properties are intricately involved with serotonin, a neurochemical involved in regulating various functions of the nervous system, including pain. Noni's xeronine system may utilize serotonin to effectively fight conditions involving chronic or excess pain.

Noni's Other
Health Benefits

WE'VE DISCUSSED FOUR major health problems—cancer, diabetes, high blood pressure, and chronic pain—which have been successfully treated using the tropical fruit noni. There are, however, many, many more that have been reported to respond positively to a health plan that utilizes noni for its incredible health benefits. The following gives a good review of some of the remaining health conditions for which noni has enjoyed popularity in treating.

Fibromyalgia and Chronic Fatigue Syndrome

If you have been diagnosed with fibromyalgia, formerly referred to as "fibrositis," "tension myalgia," or "generalized rheumatism," or chronic fatigue syndrome (CFS), also known as myalgic encephalomyelitis or the proper name "chronic fatigue and immune dysfunction syndrome (CFIDS), no one needs to tell you of the almost daily muscle pain you live with, as well as the constant fatigue, depression, sleeplessness and other symptoms that constantly plague your life. Both conditions can impart a devastating toll on previously healthy individuals, the majority of whom are women from their teens to late seventies. Not only does it strike during young and middle adult years, the busiest and most stressful time of one's life, but patients tell of how its effects make them feel as if they're 100 years old (or older!).

My study revealed some interesting findings. These showed that more than 75 percent of individuals with CFIDS became sick before the age of 50, while most became sick between their late twenties and mid-forties. Over a quarter reported that they had been sick for as long as they could remember. Fifty-five percent said they had the disease for more than five years, and about half of them remembered a "trigger" event that seemed to mark the onset of their condition. These findings were corroborated by a survey conducted by the Chronic Fatigue and Immune Dysfunction Association of America.[1]

The good news is that it does not have to be this way! There is now more knowledge than ever as to its causes and how to manage it. You can live actively with fibromyalgia and/or CFIDS, especially if a holistic health plan of diet, exercise, supplementation—including noni—and other lifestyle changes is actively employed.

Years ago, it became apparent to me and other doctors that patients who told of having muscle aches, overwhelming fatigue, depression, headaches, decreased mental abilities, and sleeplessness were in fact harboring a distinct disease or syndrome (a collection of symptoms that comprise a disease). The results from lab tests and x-rays, however, were almost always normal. Two decades ago, doctors had to send these patients home with few or no answers as to the cause of the disease or even what it was.

Today, we know differently. The past several years has brought us a rather large and impressive body of research on the mysterious and related syndromes that we call fibromyalgia and chronic fatigue and immune deficiency syndrome. Now, sufferers can understand that these diseases are real, the symptoms are not imagined or simply "in their head," and treatment, if followed faithfully, can work to help reverse the diseases' damaging effects and restore health.

The results of a recent study published in the journal *Pediatrics* showed that many children suffering from chronic fatigue and juvenile rheumatoid arthritis had psychological symptoms. But as author Bram D. Carter, M.D., and his colleagues pointed out, many of the patients studied "didn't have any psychological symptoms prior to the onset of fatigue. So the dramatic impact on their lifestyle tends to be the culprit."[2]

The findings of another recent study supported my longtime belief that persons seeking relief from symptoms of CFIDS would feel stigmatized and that the stigma was made worse when doctors attributed their symptoms to psychological causes. For that reason, 39 percent of patients with bona fide CFIDS were secretive about their symptoms in some circumstances.[3]

What is Fibromyalgia?

We all get tired. And who doesn't occasionally feel sore, achy, or stiff, especially after a weekend of sports activities or heavy gardening? For those with fibromyalgia, these debilitating symptoms are not only constant—lasting for months and years—but they are also usually much more severe, costing the patient their quality of life through ruining a career, affecting family relations and damaging their own personal life.

Gena, a fibromyalgia sufferer for over 15 years (though she was told she had fibromyalgia only 4 years ago), has experienced a widespread pain from her shoulders to the back or her neck and down to her legs. She describes the pain as "stabbing and throbbing." This forty-four-year-old woman worked full time as a data processor, but the pain had become so unbearable that she could not sit for more than ten or fifteen minutes at a time. Consequently, she had to quit. She continues:

> I used to wake up every day with stabbing pain, but thought that maybe it would go away. When I got to work and sat at the computer, the pain almost immediately began, first a dull throbbing, then increasing to a knife-like piercing. After work, I would go home, crash on the bed, and wait for it to go away. It usually didn't, so I could not cook dinner, do dishes or complete any other household chores. If my husband or children touched me, I would cringe because of the tenderness and soreness all over. And I would usually end up going to bed early—like 8:00 p.m. or so—because of being so exhausted as well in pain. But despite going to bed early, I would never sleep well and wake up tired.
>
> This went on for years until I could not stand it any more.

"I Am Completely Free From Any Medications!"

Tommy Joe Lyons, a member of the "Noni Blues" performance group, describes how noni helped him overcome his serious health problems.

"In 1983, just before my 31st birthday I was diagnosed with embryonic cell carcinoma. My prognosis for survival was not very good. In fact, many of my doctors said there was no possibility for survival. I had many surgical procedures, which included removal of the lower lobe of my left lung, a paracardiectomy (removal of the lining around the heart) and removal of a sperm cord. I was given toxic levels of chemotherapy twice, because at this point I was categorized as a stage four, which meant I had nothing to lose.

"One day a doctor walked into my room and asked if I wanted to live. I told her that not only did I want to, but that I had no doubt that I was going to live. She gave me information on a diet program called macrobiotics. Even at this time I felt that there was basis in nature to help us heal our bodies. To make a long story of numerous years of intensive medical and nutritional treatment into a short one, my cancer eventually went into remission. My body had been through hell and now was the time to heal and to recover from the residual damage of the harsh chemotherapy.

"At the time of my surgeries, it was not known that after a person receives the combination of drugs used in my chemotherapy, the body can react with fibrosis tumors in the lungs. This happened to me, and I was left with severe scarring and fibrosis tumors in my lung, partial renal failure and a depleted immune system.

"I spent the next ten years living with less than 60 percent lung capacity, battling numerous respiratory infections, fatigue, and water retention. I was so grateful to be alive that I could live with the side effects.

"In September of 1997 my singing partner, Gary Romer, talked me into trying a fruit juice called noni. I was a mainly interested in noni because I suffered from various aches and pains that were caused by heredity, arthritis and a misspent youth of intense foot-ball, baseball and basketball. (My knees, ankles and shoulders had taken a beating.)

"I was amazed that after only three weeks of drinking Tahitian Noni Juice™ I was no longer taking any pain medication for my pain and was feeling less pain than when I had been taking the medications. Also, my stomach had stopped hurting (which was a side effect from the arthritis medication). I also noticed that I didn't feel as tired. The real bonus of noni was that I went through the entire winter without even one case of bronchitis or pneumonia.

"My last lung capacity test showed that my lungs had improved to almost 90 percent of normal, and for the first time since my cancer I could qualify for life insurance. My kidney func-tion has also improved and I do not have as severe a problem with swelling in my legs and ankles.

"Sixteen years ago I was not given a chance to live. Ten years ago, although I was alive, my prospects of leading a productive and enjoyable life were nonexistent. Today, thanks to Tahitian Noni Juice™, I am a music performer with the physical stamina to travel the world, I am an avid golfer who has experienced a hole in one, and I am completely free from taking any medications. In fact, the only time there is ever a threat to my health is when I spend too much time on the golf course and I don't get the lawn mowed."

SYMPTOMS OF FIBROMYALGIA

Intense pain. Pain is the most common complaint associated with fibromyalgia, affecting about 97 percent of patients. Unlike the pain of bursitis, osteoarthritis, or tendinitis, which is usually relegated to a specific joint or area, this pain can be felt over the entire body and is "deep," sharp, dull, throbbing or aching. The pain is also usually felt in the muscles and connective tissues, rather than in the joints, though joint pain in fibromyalgia sufferers is also fairly common.

The pain can come on gradually with no apparent trigger, or can come on suddenly with or without a triggering factor, such as house-

Possible Causes of Fibromyalgia

MENOPAUSE. Some researchers suggest that the loss of estrogen, which occurs during menopause, may trigger the development of fibromyalgia. The fact that more women experience the onset of the disease between the ages of forty and fifty-five supports this theory.

SEROTONIN DEFICIENCY. Plenty of research has linked deficiencies of serotonin or its precursor, tryptophan, to the development of FMS. While still unclear, some results suggest that abnormal levels of serotonin and other substances might explain the increase in pain that patients feel. Abnormal serotonin levels may also explain some of the sleep dysfunction associated with FMS.

INFECTION, INJURY OR OTHER TRAUMA. Many patients report first feeling symptoms of fibromyalgia immediately following a significant health problem, such as an injury, a case of the flu, or following the contraction of Lyme disease. While research is still unclear, there is plenty of data in this area to support the notion that multiple factors can contribute to the incidence of FMS.

DEFICIENCY OF MINERALS, OTHER NUTRIENTS. There are researchers who strongly believe that a lack of minerals such as magnesium and other nutrients can either cause or contribute to the incidence of FMS. Health practitioners who have successfully reversed the condition in individuals attribute some of their success to the employment of dietary supplements of such nutrients.

UNDUE STRESS/EMOTIONAL TRAUMA. Mounting evidence indicates that fibromyalgia is linked to stress or emotional illness. On the other hand, some studies show that psychological stress in the patient is often very high before the disease develops. This also brings up the question as to the role the body's own biochemicals play in encouraging the onset of the syndrome.

Whatever, the cause, the vicious cycle of pain, fatigue and disturbed sleep leads to less activity, greater depression, more pain, even less sleep, more fatigue, deeper depression, and so on.

work or exercise. And it can become so intense that even prescription pain-killers won't do much to stem it. Many patients also tell of incredibly intense headaches with accompanying pain in the neck and shoulders.

Extreme fatigue. Next to the pain and overall soreness/tenderness, fatigue is the most common complaint linked with fibromyalgia. We all know what it feels like to be tired. But feeling constantly fatigued is another matter. Fibromyalgia causes a constant fatigue that limits the sufferer in her activities, whether it be work, gardening or even light house work. This fatigue can make patients say that they consistently feel tired even when they have had plenty of sleep and should feel rested. Some patients admit to feeling sleepy, though the more common complaint is that of general exhaustion without feeling drowsy or sleepy. This could be compared to having the flu or the feeling after long mental exertion.

Why is there fatigue in fibromyalgia patients? Just as the exact cause(s) of fibromyalgia is unknown, the reason that fatigue is so common is also a mystery. Sleep disturbances, common in fibromyalgia sufferers, may certainly play a part. (In fact, studies have shown that many of fibromyalgia's symptoms can be caused in otherwise healthy people if their sleep is disturbed.) Fatigue is so affecting in many patients that they would prefer to put up with the pain if their fatigue could be eliminated.

Depression. Depression is also a key symptom in fibromyalgia patients. In fact, anxiety and depression severe enough to interfere with daily activities occur in at least half of all sufferers. How does it occur? First, stress from the constant pain and fatigue can cause anxiety. The chronic pain can also lead to less physical activity, resulting in the patient becoming more withdrawn, which ultimately can bring about feelings of depression. No matter the exact cause, anxiety and depression can greatly interfere with a patient's activities at home, work and in the community.

Morning stiffness. More than three quarters of fibromyalgia sufferers feel severe stiffness in the morning upon arising. This stiffness creates a feeling of the need to loosen before beginning the day's activities. The stiffness can be extensive, spreading from the muscles and joints of the back, arms and legs. In some patients, the morning stiffness may last only a few minutes, while others experience it for significantly longer periods of time.

"Trigger" points. Many patients suffer sharp, throbbing pain that is usually accompanied by what we refer to as "trigger points," localized areas of tenderness usually around joints (though not the joints themselves) that hurt when pressed, as with a finger. These are not areas of deep pain, but rather superficial areas seemingly under the surface of the skin, such as over the elbow or shoulder.

Chronic headaches. More than half of all fibromyalgia sufferers suffer from chronic headaches. They are often caused by tightness in and contraction of the muscles of the neck and head, and are usually referred to as "tension" headaches or "muscle-contraction" headaches. They may also be caused by tenderness from trigger points over the back of the head and neck. As we have already discussed, it is important to remember that headaches can be caused by other medical problems, which should be properly diagnosed and treated.

Irritable bowel syndrome. A condition characterized by abdominal cramps and pain and periods of alternating diarrhea and constipation, irritable bowel syndrome (IBS) is found in about one-third of all fibromyalgia patients.

Menstrual cramps. Unusually painful cramps are found in 30 to 40 percent of women with fibromyalgia. It is important to note that other factors can cause a similar condition.

There are other factors that worsen symptoms; these include fatigue, changes in weather, periods of emotional stress, physical exhaustion, sedentary lifestyle, lack of sleep, feelings of anxiety and depression, smoking, excessive alcohol, and drug abuse.

SYMPTOMS OF CHRONIC FATIGUE AND IMMUNE DEFICIENCY SYNDROME

Pam, a 35-year-old mother of two, has experienced a wide assortment of symptoms resulting from chronic fatigue syndrome. She says:

> I have had CFIDS for four years, suffering through frequent headaches, severe muscle and joint pain, sleep problems, constant lethargy and fatigue, memory problems and "brain fog," frequent infections, and occasional migraines. My treatments for CFIDS have centered mainly on eliminating my symptoms. It has been a difficult four years.
>
> However, a physician friend of mine suggested that I try noni, which I did. The results were astounding. Within just three or four days, I noticed a big difference in my pain levels, my sleep had improved substantially, and I felt much more energetic. I really believe these benefits to be the result of noni because I did nothing different during that time than what I had previously been doing.

Chronic fatigue and fibromyalgia occur in varying degrees of severity. Pam's condition bordered on being severe. Many people have mild to moderate fatigue with achiness and poor sleep. Often, these people attribute the symptoms simply to aging or stress. Others have fatigue so disabling that they cannot even get out of bed, let alone participate in regular day to day activities.

When I was practicing medicine, the most common complaints that chromic fatigue patients reported to me included the following:

Overwhelming fatigue. Most people with CFIDS are fatigued most of the time. Occasionally, they have periods—that is short spans of time lasting for several hours or days during which they feel better.

Most CFIDS patients wake up tired. This is especially true of fibromyalgia patients. In addition, exercise can often make the fatigue worse. When CFIDS patients try to exercise, they feel more fatigued later that day and usually feel as if they were hit by a truck the next day. This causes further deconditioning and discouragement.

Frequent infections. Many CFIDS patients have recurrent sinus or respiratory infections, sore throats, swollen glands, bladder infections or vaginal, bowel, or skin yeast infections. Some have a recurrent red bumpy rash that is resistant to treatment. They often find that this rash goes away for the first time in years when they have their bowel fungal overgrowth treated. Abdominal gas, cramps, and bloating are also very common, as is alternating diarrhea and constipation. These digestive complaints are attributed to spastic colon and are often triggered by bowel yeast or parasitic infections. Poor food absorption and food sensitivities may also play a significant role in the onset of bowel symptoms.

Brain fog. A condition characterized by cloudy thinking and mental lethargy, "brain fog" is almost routine. Chronic fatigue patients often suffer from poor memory and occasionally from confusion. Brain fog is one of the most frustrating symptoms of CFIDS for some patients and is often the scariest.

Achiness. Chronic diffuse achiness in both muscles and joints is also very common in chronic fatigue patients. For most, this achiness is part of their fibromyalgia.

Increased thirst. When I would meet a new patient who had a water bottle in hand, I would usually know what the main complaint would be. As part of their hormonal problems, people with chronic fatigue have increased urine output and therefore increased thirst. A classic description of these patients is that they "drink like a fish and pee like a race horse." Drinking a lot of water is very important. In fact many CFIDS patients find that they need to drink two to three times as much liquids as the average person. I recommended filtered water.

Allergies. Fatigue patients often have a history of being sensitive to many foods and medications. They often get away with small doses of medications and respond adversely to normal or large doses. Fortunately, severe environmental sensitivity is much less common. I find that food and other sensitivities usually improve when the adrenal insufficiency and yeast or parasitic overgrowth are treated.

Anxiety and depression. People with CFIDS commonly have marked anxiety with palpitations, sweating and other signs of panic. The CFIDS, combined with nutritional deficiencies, aggravates the tendency to anxiety and depression.

CAUSES OF FIBROMYALGIA

Despite the fact that literally hundreds of thousands of Americans suffer from fibromyalgia, there is still no real concrete understanding of what causes it. Multiple theories abound, and recent investigation has given us more clues as to possible causes. What is becoming more apparent is that there probably is no one single cause; rather, it seems that most patients may have several contributing factors that comprise the cause of their particular condition. Moreover, these factors vary widely from patient to patient. In one it may be an emotional trauma, coupled with a bout of depression. In another, it may be one or more serious bouts of flu that mark the onset of fibromyalgia.

In this sense, then, fibromyalgia is still a sort of "mystery" condition. We basically know the symptoms and the effects. The cause, or causes, however, are clouded, which makes it all the more difficult to effectively treat the condition.

On the other hand, there are doctors and other health professionals who have developed treatment programs centered around the whole person—the physical, emotional, mental and spiritual—who have reported exciting results. Many of these programs utilize dietary supplements such as magnesium, antioxidants, calcium—and noni—to either lessen symptoms drastically or completely reverse the condition. As I have stated before, consuming noni can have spectacular results; however, it can produce even more impressive results if integrated into a lifestyle that promotes healthy eating habits, regular exercise, adequate stress relief, and proper emotional maintenance.

CAUSES OF CHRONIC FATIGUE (CFIDS)

Like fibromyalgia, the origins of CFIDS aren't exactly understood. There is plenty of research, however, that gives us some good clues as

"Keep with It"

Janeane, a real estate broker, relates how noni helped her reverse many of the fibromyalgia symptoms adversely affecting her.

"For more than five years, I ached all over, I was bone tired, and I always felt irritable and and miserable. I planned to drive to a specialist in Cleveland a few hundred miles away, but I knew I couldn't make the trip because of my misery. So, I boarded a plane and made the trip. I was then told by physicians there that I had fibromyalgia.

"Five years of pain and pills later, I felt that if my brain let go for an instant, my body would collapse as though I had no bones. My work had suffered, my social life was gone, and my family, bless them, stood by me when I didn't even like myself.

"About this time, my doctor put me on a new drug in an attempt to stop some of my pain. Soon after starting on the drug, my son found me face-down in the closet. My heart had stopped! The drug had apparently caused a lengthening of my t-waves, causing it to eventually stop. This happened three more times before the night was over. For sixty hours, until the drug could exit my system, I was critical. Then all my medications were taken away—my pain killers, my sleeping pills, my muscle relaxants, and my blood pressure medicine. I was told to take it easy and take no medications for a while. Later, though, I was again hospitalized after resuming my high blood pressure treatment.

"Soon after, a friend of mine, Joyce, called me several times, telling me about a new product that she thought could help me. She even invited me to a meeting that would explain everything I might need to know about it. But I really wasn't interested. I was simply surviving, existing. The night of the meeting came, and as I dragged myself home, my husband came out of the room dressed to go out. I asked what the occasion was, and he said he thought we should go to the meeting.

"So we did. I was miserable most of that night. I hurt sooooo bad during the meeting, and my husband and I didn't talk much on the way home. But something about the way all those people explained how noni juice had helped with this problem and that condition triggered something in me. I figured I had nothing to lose, so I called Joyce and purchased a bottle of noni juice.

"Admittedly, I was still a bit skeptical about taking the noni. Plus, I'd had some bad experiences with other medications previously, so I wasn't big on taking anything, synthetic or natural. But I finally started, taking one teaspoon twice daily, gradually increasing to a dose of one tablespoon four times daily.

"On the third morning, when I awoke, I realized that it was not the pain in my legs that awakened me, as was usually the case. I simply woke because I was rested. One month later, things had really changed for me. I have been able to drop all my medications. My fibromyalgia symptoms had virtually disappeared, leaving me almost entirely pain free. And after revisiting my cardiologist to have further testing done, he informed me that my critical markers had improved greatly. He asked if I had been doing something different. Of course, I told him about noni and the other benefits I was receiving from it. He told me to 'stick with it.'

"Noni has brought other great blessings into my life. After seeing how noni had allowed me to regain a level of relatively great health, my husband, who has had heart problems of his own, decided to begin taking noni. After just a few weeks, he says that he feels better than he has in years.

"It's incredible think that one month ago, I was skeptical about taking this 'miracle' juice. Now, I'm a believer!"

to its causes. Many believe that it is linked to the Epstein-Barr virus (EBV), a member of the herpesvirus family that is also the cause of mononucleosis. This belief is centered in the fact that many people with CFS have been found to have high levels of EBV antibodies in their blood, and that many patients date the onset of their CFS symptoms to a prolonged bout with a viral infection.

Jacob Teitelbaum, M.D., in his book, *From Fatigued to Fantastic*, also notes that many CFIDS patients report experiencing a "brutal, flulike illness that never goes away."[4] Steven Hall, M.D., a craniosacral therapist, reported to me that this is exactly what happened to one of his patients. He explained that a 55-year-old female, who three years earlier had experienced a complete recovery from a 15-year bout with chronic fatigue syndrome, once again began experiencing CFIDS symptoms after suffering from a viral infection. The good news is that Dr. Hall reported that after incorporating noni into her daily health regime for only five days, the patient improved by about 90 percent, and was currently in virtual remission.

Whether this infection is the flu or some other infection that is related, it is believed that the infection usually results in inflammation in the brain which ultimately damages the hypothalamus and pituitary gland.[5] Injury to the hypothalamus is commonly seen in CFIDS patients. What happens when the pituitary is injured? Being the body's master gland, it controls most of the other glands, including the adrenal and thyroid glands. When its function is suppressed, it in turn causes a subtle but disabling decrease in the functioning of many of the other glands. Finally, the body's various processes governed by these glands can be disrupted, manifested as the classic symptoms of chronic fatigue syndrome and/or fibromyalgia.

Other possible causes of chronic fatigue are currently under heavy investigation. Some experts point to a possible defect in the mechanisms that affect blood pressure. Others suspect anemia, chronic mercury poisoning from dental fillings, hypoglycemia, hypothyroidism, candidiasis, and sleep problems. The majority of health professionals familiar with CFIDS generally believe, however, that it is probably caused by a multitude of combinations of these and other factors.

Noni to the Rescue

Remember Gena, the data processor who had to quit her job because her fibromyalgia became so unbearable? She tried everything in the conventional treatment arsenal, including pain-killers, anti-inflammatories, and the like. She also dabbled with a few herbs and vitamin/mineral supplements. But nothing really seemed to help. Fortunately, a friend of Gena's introduced her to noni and encouraged her to try it. Gena concludes her encouraging account:

I was somewhat unbelieving. How could a fruit juice cure my problems? But I decided to try it. A few days went by, but I didn't notice anything substantial. After a week, however, I could really tell a difference. I was not sore in the mornings like usual. And the pain that started within an hour of waking up didn't come until about noon. And even then, it was not nearly as intense as before.

After about three weeks on noni, I felt like a new woman. I was experiencing almost no pain, and I had so much energy. I was going to bed around eleven or twelve instead of eight in the evening. I began gardening again, and I could take regular walks and hikes in the hills with my husband. Another great thing about it all is that I have been able to go back to work: although I occasionally need to take breaks, I am able to perform at about 200 percent of my previous capability. Noni has been a literal life-saver for me!

HOW NONI RELIEVES PAIN, FATIGUE AND OTHER PROMINENT SYMPTOMS OF FIBROMYALGIA AND CFIDS

The fact that we don't really know the exact cause or causes of fibromyalgia makes it even more difficult to assign a causative factor to noni's apparent ability to relieve its symptoms. On the other hand, there are several plausible explanations as to how and why noni can help fibromyalgia patients experience a lessening in their suffering.

First, we have previously examined how noni may enhance the body's utilization of necessary nutrients via the Golgi apparatus (GA), an irregular network of layered tubes near the nucleus of the cell. Simply stated, the principal function of the Golgi apparatus is to package and ship various compounds, such as proteins, off to other cells that need them. It is a fascinating process that resembles a very effective post office of sorts—each package is "labeled" and "delivered" to the intended cell address, after which the contents of the package is incorporated into the cell and utilized as needed.

Let's bring noni into this theory concerning the symptoms of fibromyalgia. When noni is consumed, its various components are incorporated into the body. One of these, proxeronine, travels to the cytoplasm of the body's cells and accumulates in the Golgi apparatus.

Within the GA, proxeronine combines with the other biochemicals and building blocks the body uses to help maintain efficient and properly functioning cells. These biochemicals would include hormones, proteins, enzymes, serotonin, vitamins, minerals, antioxidants, and various others. The combination of proxeronine with these other compounds are specific and varied, according to the need of the cell to which they are being sent. The Golgi apparatus then assembles the necessary ingredients into a "package," gives it a cellular "address," and delivers it via the bloodstream to the appropriate cell. As the package is opened, the proxeronine combines with a specific enzyme, proxeroninase, and is converted to xeronine. Xeronine then works with the other necessary biochemicals to create the required adaptogenic compound for that particular cell, allowing the cell to repair and regenerate itself. It is within this process that the cells regain their state of homeostasis (balance), which ultimately leads the body to an overall balanced state.

Of course, the limiting factor in this process is the proxeronine, which fortunately can be replenished by consuming adequate amounts of noni. The more "sick" or damaged a cell, the greater the amount of noni will be required to repair that cell. It is also very obvious that different cells from different organs and tissues will have specific and varying needs to both maintain normal function and to undertake any repairs it may need. In the case of the fibromyalgia sufferer, fatigue is one of the most common complaints. What causes the fatigue? As we've already mentioned, the causes aren't completely known, but it almost certainly has to do with the poor functioning of certain cells and tissues. If our body's available energy supplies are not utilized efficiently, then the individual cells can't function at optimal levels, which can ultimately lead to an overall "slowing" of the entire body. This can manifest itself in constant fatigue, unclear thinking or "brain fog," feelings of depression, and a lack of desire to complete life's normal tasks. Conversely, noni users have reported incredible success rates in treating the variety of symptoms associated with these debilitating syndromes.

Another way noni may help fight chronic fatigue and fibromyalgia is through its pain-lessening ability. As we examined in chapter 8, chronic pain, whether associated with fibromyalgia or chronic fatigue syn-

"All the Pain Was Gone!"

Tess, a registered nurse, describes her experience using noni to help relieve her symptoms of chronic fatigue syndrome:

"Four and a half years ago, I began suffering various symptoms—extreme tiredness, no energy, constant pain, sleep problems—to the point that I was eventually hospitalized. I was shortly thereafter diagnosed with chronic fatigue syndrome.

"Things were horrible. I spent several months bedridden, unable to do even the most simple household tasks. If it weren't for my husband's selflessness and doing what it took to keep things going at home, all the while working a very stressful job, I don't know what I would have done.

"During all this, I was constantly trying to find something that could help me. I had previously worked with a doctor specializing in preventive medicine, where I learned a considerable amount concerning nutrition, supplements, and alternative medicine. I was already eating well, and began trying a variety of nontraditional treatments: chelation therapy, colonics, antidepressants, antibiotics, macrobiotic diets, etc. However, these things could not really seem to help much. I felt doomed to live my life 'half alive.'

"Early this year, though, things turned around. An acquaintance of my husband told him that he had been taking noni juice, and had seen a real improvement in his chronic fatigue symptoms. Only one day later, my neighbor told me that her physician advised her to take this same noni juice for a stomach problem. She did, and after three days, her condition improved greatly. She also noticed a substantial increase in her energy levels.

"At first, I thought, 'Oh no, not another "miracle" product.' But as I thought more and more about it, I decided I had nothing to lose. So I began taking noni, and after only five days, not only did the fatigue disappear, but I had increased energy and motivation to do everything I had not been able to the last several months. And that's not all—the pain that I had constantly been feeling subsided to almost nothing.

"I am proud and delighted to add my testimony to the thousands of those who have been helped by this wonderful product, and I thank God many times a day for this wonderful blessing!"

drome, is one of today's most common health complaints. How does noni relieve pain? The fact is, there is no clear answer; however, just as in the case with fatigue, there are several theories as to noni's ability to provide dramatic relief for fibromyalgia sufferers from their debilitating pain. Some believe that the xeronine system is solely responsible for noni's ability to provide relief. Others think that noni's ability to enhance the utilization of necessary nutrients in "sick" cells may be the answer. There is also the notion that noni can thwart the development of chronic pain via its relationship with serotonin, which can aid the body in fighting pain in numerous ways.

The fact is, there probably is something to all of these theories. If we look at the xeronine system, and how it works to help "sick" or malfunctioning cells regain normal function, we can form a connection between pain and noni's apparent pain-fighting capabilities.

When considering what pain is, we know that pain is most often a symptom of an underlying cause created by the body to alert the mind to the presence of the problem. For instance, you know almost immediately that you have cut your finger because of the pain you feel. Or, you can gradually feel pain as an infection slowly develops in your lungs. In any case, pain is usually just a way for the body to alert the "intellect" that there is a problem.

So how can the xeronine system provide relief? If the body is suffering from a problem caused chiefly by the malfunction of individual cells (such as in diabetes or cancer), then noni can apparently provide needed nutrients in proper amounts to these cells, helping "repair" the condition. Thus, any pain resulting from the condition will be at least partially alleviated.

In 1992, Julia Morton, a noted botanist, reported that noni contains terpenes, found in essential oils that have been shown to aid in cell synthesis and cell rejuvenation. Other recent research reveals that noni contains numerous known essential nutrients, including proteins, amino acids, enzymes, vitamins and minerals, that may synergistically contribute to noni's ability to fight pain and a host of other ailments. I believe that the xeronine system, working principally through the Golgi apparatus, provides these nutrients to the individual cells that need them to facilitate repair and a return to optimal function.

Another way noni may help fight the pain associated with fibromyalgia and chronic fatigue disorder is through its intimate relationship with the multitalented biochemical serotonin. As we talked about in chapter 8, it is the opinion of several prominent researchers familiar with noni that it can enhance the body's utilization of serotonin. We also discussed how serotonin can specifically improve the elasticity in blood vessels and promote relaxation in abnormally constricting and relaxing muscles and blood vessels, all of which can contribute to severe and chronic pain. Dr. Khalsa, pain expert, also believes that normalizing serotonin levels in the body can help alleviate the effects of migraines by more ways than just improving the elasticity of blood vessels. These include raising the brain's pain threshold, promoting healthy sleep patterns, reducing pain-amplifying anxiety, and reducing pain-amplifying depression, all problems associated with fibromyalgia and chronic fatigue sufferers.

Recent years have expanded our knowledge of serotonin and the multiple roles it plays in relieving conditions like depression, anxiety, and sleep dysfunction. It achieves these things largely because of the role it plays in the brain and nervous system. Dr. Heinicke's extensive research revealing noni's part in the body's production and proper utilization of serotonin provides us with exciting possibilities as to how noni relieves pain. We know that serotonin, triggered by the brain, tells the nerves that first picked up the pain signal to "calm down," causing the muscles and blood vessels around the injured areas to relax. Your body loosens up, causing the pain to subside and letting you get back to feeling better.

RELIEF FROM THE PAIN, RELIEF FROM THE FATIGUE

I am amazed at noni's potent ability to relieve the debilitating effects of fibromyalgia and chronic fatigue disorder. In my survey of more than 10,000 noni users and 50 doctors and health professionals employing noni in their practice, I found that a large majority of sufferers found relief after using noni. For instance, nearly three-quarters of those taking noni to help improve their "fuzzy" thinking and mental acuity experienced positive results. Additionally, 87 percent of those taking noni to help relieve pain (including headaches) found that they were helped significantly by taking the fruit supplement. When it comes to sleep disorders (which are extremely common in fibromyalgia and chronic fatigue patients), noni has an excellent track record, helping nearly three-quarters of patients. Noni also helped relieve symptoms of depression in 77 percent of noni users, and brought about an increase of energy levels in an astounding 91 percent of those taking it.

Of course, not all of these people were necessarily suffering from fibromyalgia or chronic fatigue, though the symptoms of fibromyalgia and chronic fatigue are often similar to or intertwined with other conditions. The fact remains that tens of thousands of people, coupled with hundreds of years of folk use and a growing body of scientific research, can attest to the fact that noni not only can help reverse the progression of fibromyalgia and chronic fatigue syndrome, but a wide array of other health conditions as well.

Arthritis

Some people mix up osteoarthritis and rheumatoid arthritis, two very different rheumatologic diseases with similar names. And it gets even more confusing when you learn there are more than 100 different types of rheumatic diseases, many causing different forms of "arthritis."[6] For the reason that many readers may be confused by a separation of the various forms of arthritis, I have included a short description of causes, symptoms and other commentary of each condition that falls under the blanket term "arthritis."

Despite the occasional confusion as to what arthritis is and isn't, the fact remains that millions of people world wide suffer from one form of arthritis or the other. Marion was one of these people. She experienced some of the most typical symptoms of arthritis, but most notably a constant, dull pain in her back that limited her physical activity. She explains:

For years, I have suffered from arthritic pain in my back. At one point it was so bad that I had to roll very slowly out of bed and use the furniture next to the bed to even stand up. Of course, there were a number of things that I could not do around the house, including gardening and yard work. Not long ago, I was introduced to noni by a friend, who explained all of its wonderful health benefits. So I began taking it.

Within about three weeks of taking the noni juice, the severe pain in my back had nearly vanished, and I could rise from bed or a sitting position with little complaint from my back. I became so happy that I went to my good friend's house and pranced about her kitchen, excitedly yelling, "Can you believe this?" My arthritis has improved so much that I have been out raking leaves with my daughter, I have again started jogging, and I have even shoveled snow—something I had not done in years.

I've had other problems as well, especially with digestion, that have been cleared up using noni. I have long prayed that I could find an answer to my arthritis and other problems. My prayers have definitely been answered because I can eat just about anything I want and I am pain free!

Marion's type of arthritis was limited mainly to the joints in her back, and manifested itself principally in severe and long-lasting pain. Depending upon the type of arthritis, the associated inflammation, tenderness and pain may flare up in one joint or many, may limit itself to the joint only, or might spread to the muscles, tendons, ligaments, internal organs, and even the skin. Different types of arthritis have different causes, symptoms and courses. A competent health professional can help diagnose what type of arthritis you may have, which may very well be one of these common forms.

How noni combats the various forms of arthritis, connective tissue problems and related conditions are discussed in other sections of this book.

"I'm a Much Happier Person to Be Around!"

Toni, a 54-year-old woman, describes her experience with noni:

"I'm a grandmother of nine children, with a body that has been slowly falling apart. I have had numerous health problems for many years now, many resulting from my being overweight. The most terrible of all my problems was arthritis, which at times became so bad that every move I made was rewarded with excruciating pain. For years I took all kinds of medications, but they all made me sick or didn't really work.

"Besides the pain, I had to have total knee replacement on my right knee due to the cartilage becoming so damaged because of the arthritis. I've also suffered from high blood pressure, diabetes, asthma, sleep apnea, and chronic fatigue syndrome. I was on a number of pills for these problems, all of which caused me to have problems sleeping, as well as a number of unwanted side effects.

"In July, I was visiting my family in Indiana. My sister and mother began to tell me I should try a particular new product, and about how it had helped them with a number of health problems. At first I declined, but after several pain-filled days there, I relented and began taking the noni juice. It was one of the best decisions I've ever made.

"Some time after starting on noni, I went in to see my doctor because of a car accident I was in. He had not seen me for a few months, and he noticed a big difference in my overall health right away. He ran several tests, and commented that my blood pressure was much better, my skin color was more normal, and the bruising from the accident had healed much quicker than anticipated. He also inquired about my daily fatigue, and I was able to tell him that it was gradually getting better.

"Today, I am not taking anything for pain, and I don't need to use my cane much at all to walk. One of the biggest blessings is that I'm also able to keep up with my grandkids, who live close. An added bonus has been my losing 20 pounds (for the first time in 30 years), which will also help with most of my problems.

"Noni has been a huge blessing. I have more energy, my arthritis is nearly gone, I handle stress much better, and I sleep much better at night. In the end, I am a much happier person to be around."

OSTEOARTHRITIS

Though the literal translation of the word *osteoarthritis* means "inflammation of the bone joint," this doesn't quite accurately describe what osteoarthritis is. Joint pain rather than inflammation is its most important characteristic. While severe inflammation is a major part of many other forms of arthritis, it is not found in most cases of osteoarthritis.

Osteoarthritis is just one of many forms of joint disease; however, it is by far the most common form, affecting articular cartilage, the smooth, bluish white substance covering the end of both bones in a joint. Over time, the wear and tear of your bones rubbing together dries out the cartilage, making it crack and deteriorate. Of course, if it becomes very severe, the cartilage can completely disappear, leaving the bone ends completely exposed. This causes a number of symptoms, including most notably pain, stiffness, a cracking/crunching sensation, deformity of the joint, and occasionally severe inflammation.

ANKYLOSING SPONDYLITIS

If you wake up in the morning with lower back pain and stiffness, if sitting or lying down for more than a couple of hours make your back feel worse, if your chest hurts when you inhale, and if you're tired and losing weight, you may be suffering from ankylosing spondylitis (AS), an autoimmune condition in which your body's own antibodies attack healthy cells.

Causing bent or fused spine vertebrae, AS is most commonly seen in young men. It sometimes goes untreated in earlier stages because it can easily be confused with simple mechanical back pain, the kind you get from lifting a heavy object. With AS, the tendons and ligaments that make it possible to move the back become inflamed. In response, the vertebrae produce more bone. Though well intentioned, the body's response of making extra bone can cause the vertebrae to grow into each other and fuse together. Eventually, the spine can wind up looking like a bamboo pole, and it bends forward under the weight of the head. If you have ever seen an elderly person walking bent over as though he were looking at his shoes, you have probably witnessed the late stages of AS.

AS inflammation usually begins in the lower back, and almost always involves the sacroiliac joints (the joints where the lower spine meets the pelvis). In later stages the middle and upper back are afflicted. The disease can spread down into the buttocks and thighs, or up into the chest, where it can make deep breathing painful. The inflammation may also strike the joints of the shoulders, knees, or ankles. In fact, in some 20 percent of AS cases the first signs of arthritis appear in the shoulder, hip, or other joints. But most of the time the disease is confined to the lower back and is relatively mild. People with AS are not usually disabled and don't have shortened careers or life spans.

BURSITIS AND TENDINITIS

Many an unhappy weekend athlete is familiar with bursitis and/or tendinitis, that pain and tenderness in the shoulders, elbows, knees, or pelvis that spreads to the nearby limbs, and is often accompanied by fever. Bursitis/tendinitis are the most common forms of soft tissue rheumatic syndromes, usually caused by the sudden overuse of a joint.

Bursa means purse, and the small fluid-filled sacs (bursae) that cushion various parts of the joints do look something like little purses. There are dozens of them in the body; each knee has eight or more. The bursae, which act as cushions (usually between soft tissue and a bony prominence), may become inflamed if a joint is subjected to abnormal pressure. This is most often the result of overuse, a chronic condition, or a traumatic injury such as a fall on the knee or elbow. The bursae can fill with more fluid than usual, triggering inflammation and pain.

Tendinitis is often grouped with bursitis, but is a very different problem. Tendinitis is characterized by the inflammation or irritation of a tendon, the tough, fibrous tissue that ties muscles to bones. We normally think that bones move only when muscles contract, but remember that the tendon is "between" the muscle and the bone, allowing the two to function together. Contracting a muscle to move a bone means that the tendons automatically "move" as well. Forcing swollen tendons to move, however, can be quite painful.

Tendinitis usually strikes suddenly. It's typically localized (restricted to one area), and can linger for days or weeks before disappearing. Many of us will have tendinitis at one time or another in our lives, but fortunately, permanent damage or disability from this condition is rare. It may strike the outside of the elbow as "tennis elbow," the inside of the elbow as "golfer's elbow," the tendons that move the fingers, the bottom of the pelvis, or the finger joints.

Bursitis and tendinitis usually occur after age 30, the result of wear and tear on the bursae and/or tendons, abnormal stress on joints or tendons, overly ambitious workouts by "weekend warriors," or a sudden strain, such as lifting a heavy package. "Bursitis/tendinitis are usually not chronic conditions, and permanent damage is rare. Noni has been reported to help with both conditions.

GOUT

In gout, uric acid, a waste product in the urea (urine) formation cycle, is either overproduced, underexcreted, or both. When a person has too much uric acid in his or her system, some of it forms uric acid crystals. These crystals can be deposited into the joint space, rather than being cleared by the kidneys. These "glass shards" often find their way to the bunion joint of the big toe, although gout is also found in the other joints of the feet, as well as those of the fingers, wrists, elbows, knees, and ankles. The afflicted joint suddenly becomes hot, painfully swollen, and stiff; fever and chills sometimes follow. The skin of the affected area can appear shiny red or purple, and pain from an acute attack of gout can be excruciating. In some cases, the joint is so tender that the light brush of a bed sheet can cause howls of pain.

Gout affects about two million Americans, most of them male (80 percent). Risk factors for getting the disease include a family history of gout, an excess of "rich" protein foods, drinking alcohol, high blood pressure, taking certain medications, being overweight, or suddenly gaining weight. Unchecked, gout can be hazardous to your health, for the uric acid crystals may eventually be deposited in the soft tissue, cartilage, joints, tendons, or elsewhere, forming lumps. The crystals can also damage the kidneys.

INFECTIOUS ARTHRITIS

Can arthritis be brought about by "germs?" Absolutely. Many forms of bacteria, viruses, and fungi can cause infectious arthritis, which is frequently characterized by loss of joint function, fever, and inflammation of one or more joints and (occasionally) chills. The knee is most commonly involved (50 percent of the cases), followed by the hip, shoulder, wrist, and ankle. Infectious arthritis can generally be effectively treated if caught early enough.

Practically any bacterium, virus, or fungus that produces disease can prompt this infectious form of arthritis, and there are many ways that the infecting agent can enter the body: trauma, surgery, sexual contact with an infected individual, inserting a needle into a joint, abscess or bone infection near the joint, animal bites, insect bites (Lyme disease), and even thorns. A less obvious but common source of joint infection is bacteria from a distant site in the body that travels through the bloodstream before settling in a joint. Infections almost anywhere in the body can move to the joints, including infections that begin in the lungs, genitals, urinary tract, and skin. Remember that any invasive procedure involving a joint (surgery, injection into the joint space) can lead to infection and infectious arthritis. This is an important consideration when opting for certain arthritis treatments that involve injecting medicine directly into the joint.

The body responds to the infection by mobilizing the immune system to battle with the infectious agent. The joint becomes the battleground. Like all battlegrounds, the joint suffers, becoming inflamed and painful as the body releases enzymes that inadvertently degrade the cartilage as they seek to destroy the invaders. Chronic alcoholics and drug abusers are at high risk for infectious arthritis, as are those suffering from diabetes, sickle cell anemia, kidney disease, certain forms of cancer, and sexually transmitted diseases.

RHEUMATOID ARTHRITIS

Rheumatoid arthritis (RA) is an autoimmune disease brought about when the body has literally started to turn on itself, with the immune system attacking bodily tissues just as if they were foreign invaders. In its mildest form, rheumatoid arthritis is characterized by joint discomfort; in its most serious form it can cause extreme pain, deformed joints and harm organ systems.

Some experts believe that RA is brought about by a bacterial infection in the joints. It might also be triggered by a virus settling in those who are genetically susceptible, causing the joint lining (especially the part that meets the cartilage) to become inflamed. Over time, chronic inflammation makes the joint lining thick and overgrown. This overgrown lining may then start to invade the cartilage, other joint-supporting tissues, and even the bone, weakening the entire joint structure. Eventually, the weakened joint becomes more painful and less able to perform. Under pressure, it may even become dislocated and deformed.

Usually appearing in the same joint on both sides of the body (both hands, for example), RA generally hits with suddenness. The joints become swollen, tender, and inflamed. This is exactly what happened with Phil, a cattle rancher suffering from inflamed and extremely sore hand joints. Having worked for years on a ranch, Phil suffered from not only arthritis, but also other aches and pains as well. He says, "I am writing this to tell about an amazing discovery that has helped my family, myself, and even my cattle. I began taking noni juice, and within days, my lower back pain disappeared. I also had arthritis in my hands, which were very sore and swollen in the mornings. After taking noni for only a few short weeks, that soreness and inflammation are now gone!"

Other symptoms of rheumatoid arthritis include fever, weight loss, and a general feeling of sickness, soreness, stiffness, and aching. The eyes and mouth may dry out if the tear and salivary glands become involved.

About 10 percent of those affected with the disease have a single episode followed by a spontaneous long-term remission. For the other 90 percent, joint inflammation is chronic, although mild, with occasional attacks or "flares." The disease may get progressively worse over time.

SYSTEMIC LUPUS ERYTHEMATOSUS

Though not a true form of arthritis, lupus, or SLE, is an autoimmune disease that attacks and inflames connective tissues throughout
the body and damages many of the body's organs. Its victims may have
a red "butterfly" rash spread across the bridge of their noses and
cheeks. The rash resembles markings on wolves, which explains the
name of the disease (*lupus* is Latin for *wolf*).

Affecting nine times as many women as men, lupus usually strikes
during the childbearing years (18 to 45) and is found in about one out
of two thousand people. The disease causes the production of abnormal antibodies called antinuclear antibodies (ANA) that damage bodily tissues. The skin, kidneys, nervous system, muscles, lungs, and
heart can all be affected, as well as the joints. Besides the red rash on
the face, common symptoms include joint pain, stiffness, fever, muscle ache, weight loss, loss of hair, and exhaustion. There may also be a
sensitivity to ultraviolet light, with exposure to the sun worsening the
rash. As the disease progresses, inflammation of the linings of the
heart, lungs, and kidneys can cause permanent damage.

As with scleroderma (tightening of the skin) and rheumatoid arthritis, an unknown trigger may set lupus in motion, but only in those who
are already genetically susceptible. The degree of severity of the disease varies quite a bit from person to person. Some don't even know
they have it and require no treatment at all, while for others it is a
major illness. The majority of people, however, have moderate symptoms and function quite well.

HOW NONI ALLEVIATES THE EFFECTS OF ARTHRITIS AND SIMILAR CONDITIONS

Of the hundreds of individuals whose feedback I received explaining how noni helped fight arthritis, there are a number of dramatic
accounts describing noni's powerful antipain and anti-inflammatory
effects. One such person, Bootsie H., provides one of these accounts:

Twenty years ago, I was diagnosed with both osteoarthritis and rheumatoid arthritis. As a result, I have been on numerous medications, including gold shots, large doses of prednisone, methotrexate, and others. Despite some relief offered by these things, their side effects often outweighed their benefits. These side effects included spastic colon, spastic bowels and bleeding of the gums. But, to get any relief from the pain, I had to endure them.

How bad was my arthritis? I could not close my hands, nor could I clap them. I had to have eleven operations on my feet because of the arthritis. In fact, I have had so many problems with arthritis in my feet and legs that I have often needed crutches or a cane to even walk. Jerry, my husband, has told me numerous times that I have cried in my sleep because of the pain.

Not long ago, I found out about the tropical fruit noni and its reported health benefits. After using it for about three weeks, I didn't notice much of a difference. However, one of the girls at the church I volunteer at asked me what I had been doing to my hands because they did not look as red or swollen as they had in the past. Taking encouragement from this, I increased my dosage of noni, and about two weeks later, my gums stopped bleeding (and they haven't bled since).

Soon, there were noticeable differences in my arthritis. Upon visiting my rheumatologist, he said he had not seen me look so well in the twenty years he had been treating me. Because of this, he was able to cut my medications by about 75 percent. The swelling in my hands is no longer there. I can close them and clap them. I also have had an enormous jump in energy that has been so dramatic that I can work an eight- to ten-hour day, cooking for more than 100 people, at my church. And I still have extra energy at the end of the day!

Like Bootsie, thousands of arthritis sufferers have found relief from the pain, inflammation and other dreadful effects of arthritis and related disorders after using noni. Like we have seen in earlier chapters of this book, pain is one of the most common complaints reported to doctors, whether it be a symptom of an underlying disease, like arthritis, or a chronic condition. Traditionally, treating pain resulting from arthritis or other related disorders has been marginally successful,

212 / THE NONI PHENOMENON

with the use of powerful prescription drugs being the principal treatment. While they may alleviate the pain and inflammation, they also usually bring a number of side effects with them.

But there are other ways of effectively finding relief from arthritis. There is powerful evidence that noni can help individuals suffering from osteoarthritis, rheumatoid arthritis, lupus, fibromyalgia, and other related disorders to alleviate their pain and inflammation and regain a state of normality in their lives. For instance, my survey of over 10,000 noni users revealed that 80 percent of more than 650 arthritis sufferers experienced a lessening of their symptoms (principally pain and inflammation) and that it enhanced the action of their current arthritis medications and/or allowed for a reduction in the doses of those medications. Other patients suffering from related conditions (i.e., bursitis, tendinitis, lupus, fibromyalgia) also reported a fantastic success rate in treating pain (see chapter 8 for more information). One such case involved Julia, a grandmother of twins, who developed tendinitis after watching her granddaughters full-time. Her arms would ache so badly that it would keep her up at night and disrupt her sleep. She tried a number of anti-inflammatories and pain-killers with no results. After taking noni for only one week, one to two ounces a day, the pain completely disappeared. She also has two degenerated discs in her neck which have affected her sleep for more than five years. After the noni treatment, the pain and discomfort in her neck has subsided, letting her sleep soundly through the night.

So how does noni help fight arthritis? While there is no definitive scientific proof, I believe that noni works via the proxeronine bundles sent by the Golgi apparatus in our cells to the specific cells and tissues suffering from the constant pain and inflammation, whether from rheumatoid arthritis, lupus or ankylosing spondylitis. For more specific information on this, see chapter 8, which deals with noni and chronic pain.

Infection from Bacteria, Viruses, Parasites and Fungi

Pathogenic invaders, such as bacteria, viruses, fungi and parasites, are responsible for a multitude of our most common health complaints. From the common cold to flesh-eating bacteria to HIV, these tricky and sometimes deadly invaders pose a very real threat to our health and well-being.

In response to this threat, people through the ages have looked for effective ways to fight infection. As we have mentioned earlier, noni has been used for centuries for various health problems, including infections, by numerous cultures worldwide.

Botanist Julia Morton explains that noni has been used in the Philippines as a vermifuge (an agent that aids the body in expelling parasites) and for relieving such conditions as boils, carbuncles and stomach ulcers (which are often caused by the bacteria *H. pylori*) in Hawaii.[7] She also notes that noni was used to treat ringworm, boils, ulcers, wounds, and as a potent insecticidal wash. Numerous other historical accounts back noni's ability to fight bacterial and viral invaders. From Guam to India to the West Indies, noni has been used to treat infected ulcers, wounds, boils, skin diseases, sinus infections, and other problems caused or exacerbated by infection.

Modern research supports the historical use of noni as an antimicrobial agent. In 1950, researchers in the journal *Pacific Science* reported that noni fruit possessed antibacterial properties against several bacterial strains: *P. aeruginosa, M. pyrogenes* and *E. coli.*[8] University of Hawaii researcher Oscar Levand also found noni fruit extract to have remarkable abilities to ward off infection from several bacterial species, including *Salmonella typhosa, Pseudomonas aeruginosa, Proteus morganii, Staphylycoccus aureus, Bacillus subtilis* and *Escherichia coli (E. coli).*[9] Furthermore, my survey of more than 10,000 noni users and 50 health professionals who suggested and/or used noni as a health supplement found that noni was very effective in treating a wide range of infections. I received literally hundreds of reports of using noni to fight abscesses and mouth/gum infections, to

214 / THE NONI PHENOMENON

"They Can't Believe What It Looks Like Now"

William describes another remarkable incident where noni was able to quickly and effectively clear up an infection.

"My wife and I were first introduced to noni by our son, who took it upon himself to drive 500 miles to personally deliver to us what he thought of as a valuable health-promoting agent. Immediately, we began drinking one ounce of the juice per day, and soon increased the amount to two ounces.

"I had taken noni for about six months when I suffered a pretty nasty cut on my wrist. I am a groundsman for a tree trimmer, and one day while trimming trees, a branch took an awkward bounce, with the cut end of the branch smashing into my wrist and leaving an open gouge wound more than one inch in diameter.

"Right away, I covered the wound with a compress soaked in noni juice. I changed the compress continually, using noni juice and occasionally hydrogen peroxide in the compress. In addition to the noni juice, I also used a noni skin product. Sometimes a bandage was used with either the juice or the skin product, or both. At other times, the skin product was applied directly to the open wound. From time to time, we would replace the noni juice in the compress with a medicine dropper.

"One immediate result of using noni was the absence of a scab. Soon, the wound closed up and healed quickly. Friends of mine who had seen the fresh wound tell me they can't believe what it looks like now. There remains only a slightly pink triangular area about half the size of the wound. I wouldn't even call it a scar."

treat colds, flu and other forms of upper respiratory tract infections, to relieve symptoms of urinary tract infections, to speed the healing of wounds, boils, ulcers and infected burns, and to battle against the detrimental effects of parasites. Interestingly, many noni juice users who were on antibiotics for bacterial infections found that noni improved their healing process.

One such story, which I received from a woman named Maren,

explained how her eight-year-old niece had been suffering from chronic bladder infections. Things had become so bad that her doctor decided to put her on a low-dose antibiotic for a few months. This troubled the girl's parents, so they decided to start giving her noni. On a Sunday they gave her one tablespoon of noni juice, and followed with a similar dose for the next four days. On Thursday, the doctor took another blood test, which yielded a negative result. Furthermore, the girl's symptoms were almost entirely absent. She has been taking noni consistently ever since, and has had no problems with her bladder infections.

Other research gives us clues as to how noni may work to fight infection. In chapter 5, we discussed in depth a study from researchers at the University of Hawaii showing that noni stimulates the production of various immune agents, including nitric oxide, interleukin 1, interleukin 2, interleukin 4, interleukin 10, interleukin 12, interferon, and lipopolysaccharide, most of which help fight many pathogens, whether they be viral, bacterial, cancerous, parasitic, or fungal.[10] Another recent study also indicates that scopoletin, a health-promoting agent found in noni, may inhibit the activity of *E. coli*, commonly associated with recent outbreaks resulting in hundreds of serious infections and even death.[11]

These and other studies provide exciting data indicating that noni can indeed aid the body in stimulating and strengthening its various immune functions, thereby adding valuable protection against pathogenic agents like bacteria, viruses, cancerous cells, fungi and parasites. Noni's principal method of helping defend against these infectious agents is its immunostimulatory ability. In other words, noni possesses the ability to stimulate or encourage the production, even above normal levels, of the already listed immune fighting cells. In turn, these cells are the primary force behind ridding the body of unwanted invaders.

"Her Family Can't Believe This Is Happening!"

Dr. John Mike has used noni to treat a variety of conditions with his patients. He explains how noni helped an elderly patient receive quick relief from foot ulcers. He explains:

"I have had many positive experiences with my patients as a result of recommending noni, but the most remarkable occurred with an elderly, wheelchair-bound woman suffering from Alzheimer's, vision problems and severe leg and foot lesions. Her podiatrist, who was treating the lesions, told this patient's niece that he was afraid that the ulcers, which weren't healing, may contribute to the spread of infection to her bones.

"As I was seeing this woman mainly for her anxiety, I recommended she start taking noni (I was hoping it would help with more than just her anxiety). After about three weeks of treatment, she visited her podiatrist for a check-up. After unwrapping her feet, the podiatrist asked the niece what she had been doing. Afraid that things were worse, the niece replied she hadn't done anything. Instead of telling them that the lesions had worsened, he informed them that the ulcers were about 90 percent healed. The doctor was extremely surprised, seeing that the ulcers were not responding to any previously prescribed treatment. The niece then informed him about her aunt taking noni, and he was very impressed, asking to get more information on it.

"About seven weeks later, I saw the elderly woman again. She had made incredible strides in other areas as well. She was spontaneously speaking and laughing, she could more clearly see images and colors, and she placed her feet on the ground and tried to stand for the first time in years. Her niece and other family members can't believe this is happening—they believe that it's literally a miracle!"

"Needless to Say, I Was Ecstatic!"

Lonnie, an HIV patient, provides a powerful account of how noni could aid AIDS patients.

"I have an incredible story to tell. I have been HIV positive since 1989. With good fortune on my side, I have been asymptomatic, and have never had to take any AIDS drugs. However, in 1996, it looked like my good luck was running out. My T-cell count had been taking a big turn downward, slipping into the 400 range, then the 300 range, in which AIDS drug therapy is strongly recommended.

"About two months after my last test, I began taking noni, a 'miracle from paradise,' on the recommendation of a friend. She said it would also help speed the healing from an upcoming surgery on my heel.

"The next day, I took my usual HIV test. Two weeks later, I took another test. That day, the doctor called to tell me he was concerned that if the results of this test turned out to be the same as or lower than the results of the test two weeks earlier, he would strongly recommend going on the drug therapy.

"Two days later, the head of the research center called to give me the 'great news'! My last test revealed that my T-cell count had jumped to 482 (it had gone down to 369), and that my ratio had risen to 41 percent. Needless to say, I was ecstatic!"

Animal and Pet Health

Though secondary to helping humans fight various health conditions, noni has also been shown to be effective in aiding animals to battle a multitude of disorders and diseases. Historical island accounts suggest that it was common for pigs to eat noni in the wild, and that those pigs who ate noni were healthier and had more stamina than animals that did not. Dr. Gary Tran, a veterinarian graduate from Oklahoma State University and staff at the Animal Emergency Center in Kentucky, who has treated over 5,000 animals with noni juice, reports that the response of most animals to noni is as good or better than their human counterparts.

Dr. Tran first heard about noni about three years ago, and was skeptical of its effectiveness. Finally, he decided to try it. The day he made the decision to try noni as a dietary supplement, his aunt called and told him that her daughter was dying of AIDS. Dr. Tran sent noni to his aunt that very day. He reports that noni helped his cousin so much that he decided to give it to his immediate family. It helped his wife's chronic fatigue syndrome and depression, as well as his son's debilitating migraine headaches. It even eased his own arthritis pain and asthma.

CONDITIONS REPORTED TO RESPOND TO NONI	# WHO TOOK NONI FOR THAT CONDITION	% HELPED
Cancer, lessened symptoms	847	67%
Heart disease, decreased symptoms	1,058	80%
Stroke	983	58%
Diabetes, Types 1 and 2	2,434	83%
Energy, increased	7,931	91%
Sexuality, enhanced enjoyment	1,545	88%
Muscle, increased body-building	709	71%
Obesity, lost excess weight	2,638	72%
High blood pressure, decreased	721	87%
Smoking, stopped	447	58%
Arthritis, lessened symptoms	673	80%
Pain, incl. headaches, decreased	3,785	87%
Depression, lessened symptoms	781	77%
Allergy, decreased symptoms	851	85%
Digestion, improved	1,509	89%
Breathing, improved	2,727	78%
Sleep, improved	1148	72%
Fuzzy thinking, helped clear	301	89%
Well-being, increased feeling of	3,716	79%
Mental acuity, increased alertness	2,538	73%
Kidney health, improved	2,127	66%
Stress, helped cope with	3,273	71%

Table 9.1: **Conditions helped by people who used noni juice (n=>10,000).** *This table depicts the pooled percentage of people who experienced objective and/or subjective improvement of their symptoms after taking noni. The majority of noni users who did not get optimal results failed to do so because they took a smaller amount and/or took it for a shorter time than what was recommended, or simply did not respond for unknown reasons.*

It should be noted that noni can be used together with all other medications because there are virtually no negative interactions. In some situations, noni can allow other medications to act more efficiently. You should tell your health professional that you are taking noni as your physician might want to decrease the dose of the medication prescribed. It should also be noted that side effects were minimal. Less than 5 percent had loose bowel movements, a slight belch or developed a mild rash. The belch and loose bowel movements disappeared when the dose was decreased. The rash cleared within 72 hours after the person stopped taking noni. Concerning use by pregnant or nursing women, noni has been reported to be safe.

The results were so dramatic for his entire family that Dr. Tran decided to use it on the four-legged patients at his clinic. He reported that more than 90 percent of the 5,000 animals have responded very positively. He notes that "noni is not only wonderful for alleviating pain, it's also antihistaminic, anthelmintic (rids animals of worms), anti-inflammatory, analgesic, and anti-carcinogenic." He believes that, like in humans, it strengthens the animal's immune system, enabling it to fight viral, bacterial and other infections. He further believes that noni heals and rejuvenates sick tissue, controls vomiting, counteracts poisons, and stabilizes animals that are in shock. It also takes care of the inflammation associated with joint problems, arthritis, sprains, and fractures. He further believes that noni helps organs to heal more quickly, reverses some neurological disorders, helps spinal cord injuries, and enables animals to come out of comas faster. Dr. Tran now rarely resorts to the use of painkillers, muscle relaxants, or steroids on most of his animal clients. Instead, he uses noni juice.

Dr. Tran cites some dramatic cases of animals being helped by noni juice. One owner accidentally ran over his dog because it was sleeping under the car, leaving the dog hobbled with several severe fractures. Dr. Tran set the broken bones in a cast and gave the dog a daily dosage of noni juice. In two weeks, the animal had completely healed. He believes the healing took place much faster because he used noni.

Another dog had been hit by a car and was suffering from severe internal injuries. Dr. Tran could not surgically repair the dog's internal injuries because of their severity. Instead, he started the dog on a regimen of intravenous fluids and noni juice by mouth. The dog's condition stabilized very quickly; consequently, Dr. Tran decided to operate. When he cut the dog open, he was astounded when he saw that many of the dog's most important internal organs had been ruptured, but were now under repair. The dog, according to Dr. Tran, surely should have been dead. Dr. Tran believes that noni helped to save the dog, which eventually made a complete recovery.

Dr. Tran notes: "I have found that noni juice is the most wonderful substance which a doctor can use in this line of work. In all my 35 years of practicing traditional and holistic veterinary medicine, I haven't seen any other product that is as versatile as noni juice. If I were banished to a remote island and could bring only one health product, it would definitely be noni juice."[12]

Proper Digestion and Elimination

After reviewing the feedback that I received from the many noni users responding to my survey, it was quite apparent that consuming noni helped promote healthy digestion. Sometimes, specific digestive disorders were reversed or alleviated, and in other cases, normalization of digestion was the result. Interested in how noni could normalize the function of the digestive tract, I soon discovered that the noni fruit contains a substantial amount of both soluble and insoluble fiber, which could account for at least some of its ability to promote a healthy digestive and eliminatory tract.

The last two centuries have brought a wealth of information concerning the role dietary fiber plays in preventing disease and enhancing overall health. Literally hundreds of studies have shown that adequate consumption of fiber can reduce the risk of various types of cancer, relieve the effects of diabetes, eliminate constipation, hemorrhoids and other related conditions, and promote a healthy cardiovascular system.

There are two types of fiber—soluble fiber, which dissolves or breaks down in water, and insoluble fiber, which does not dissolve in water. Both types of fiber are essential to good health, aiding the body in maintaining a proper weight, lowering cholesterol, promoting proper digestion and elimination, normalizing bowel movements and cleansing and promoting the growth of friendly intestinal flora. Noni contains equal proportions of soluble and insoluble, both of which contribute to various health benefits. Of course, lack of dietary fiber has been linked to a substantial number of diseases and disorders, including heart disease, appendicitis, diverticulitis, obesity, colorectal cancer, hemorrhoids, indigestion and varicose veins.

What is exciting about noni and fiber is that there are now available fiber products centered primarily around a high-fiber noni content.

Considering the many health benefits of noni fruit juice, these noni-fiber products represent a fantastic alternative to traditional fiber products.

Like many others who reported that noni helped normalize bowel function and improve digestive disorders, Kate discovered just how valuable noni could be because of its ability to alleviate symptoms of digestive distress. She explains:

> The first thing I noticed after starting to take noni juice happened about ten days into my program. I had just eaten some foods that previously, I would have stayed away from because they typically made me "pay for it." Generally, after eating foods like this, I would get fairly severe indigestion, intestinal gas and often diarrhea. However, much to my surprise, nothing happened. And it was no fluke. I have no longer had to rely on Maalox or Tagamet after eating because of what noni has done for me!

Chapter Summary Points

- Noni can provide extensive relief for sufferers of fibromyalgia, chronic fatigue syndrome and related disorders. It can help alleviate the symptoms of chronic pain, overwhelming fatigue, tendency to infections, stiffness, inflammation, "brain fog," depression, and headaches.
- A large majority of noni users that reported their cases to me experienced a relief of symptoms common to fibromyalgia and chronic fatigue syndrome after using noni.
- Noni has also enjoyed immense popularity as a treatment for the various types of arthritis: osteoarthritis, rheumatoid arthritis, gout, tendinitis, bursitis, infectious arthritis, and related conditions.
- My survey of more than 10,000 noni users and health professionals revealed that over 80 percent of the 716 patients taking it to alleviate the effects of their arthritis reported that it did just that.
- Noni probably helps relieve the symptoms of arthritis and related conditions by virtue of the proxeronine "bundles" packaged and sent by the Golgi apparatus to the affected cells and tissues.

- Plenty of historical data, as well as current research, gives validity to the notion that noni can help fight infection from various sources through stimulating the immune system. Research shows that noni enhances the immune system's ability to fight foreign invaders.
- Another popular use of noni has been for the health care of animals. I have received notice of literally thousands of cases where noni was used to successfully treat animals for a variety of conditions, ranging from wounds to arthritis to digestive disorders.

The Power of Noni

THIS BOOK IS my attempt to completely and succinctly outline the apparent health benefits of noni. Despite the fact that the body of bona fide research concerning noni's therapeutic effects is still relatively small, there is still the powerful and overwhelming effect of the tens of thousands of individuals who can attest to noni's potent health-promoting capabilities. In previous chapters, you can find ample numbers of testimonies from patients regarding how noni helped their specific condition. This chapter contains several more accounts of individuals whose stories may not have necessarily fit into one of the previous chapters, but which merit your attention. Some are incredible, others are heart-warming, but most importantly, all of these convincing accounts convey what these and other noni users have discovered. That is, noni is a safe and effective health supplement capable of providing relief from a multitude of health conditions.

"I Was Now on My Death Bed"

Kevin details his powerful account of how noni helped him literally regain his life:

"People say you don't appreciate what you have until you lose it. That was certainly true for me after a devastating fall turned my life upside down. I had a ladder collapse below me, sending me hurtling to a concrete floor from nine feet. I hit the floor with my back and my head, which left me in agonizing pain. This resulted in a protruding disc and bone contusions which disabled me for seven months. All the time I was lying in my bed unable to work and with no income, losing everything I owned. I suffered from depression and I started getting anxiety attacks, which resulted in me being rushed to the hospital several times. I was on five different prescription medications, of which a couple were addictive and which I would probably be on for the rest of my life.

"One Sunday morning, with massive pain in my chest, I called to my teenage son to rush me to the hospital. On the way, I was losing my breath and my sight and believing it to be my last day on earth. I had come to the realization that I was not going to see my son, Evan, again, and I could see him fading away from me as I sat in the seat beside him. Hardly being able to speak yet trying to say goodbye to my son was the hardest thing I have ever done. When we reached the hospital my son had to help me into the Emergency Room because I could not walk, talk or even see, and was gasping desperately for every breath. They rushed me in and worked on me for six hours, and as I lay there thinking of what had transpired I could only cry.

"This seemed to be the culmination of twenty years of suffering. In addition to the problems from my fall, I suffered from debilitating migraine headaches, and as a result of being struck by lightning, my nervous system was scrambled, leaving areas of my body numb. I was now, I thought, on my death bed.

"Despite my thinking that I didn't have much time to live, I was able to semi-recover and eventually leave the hospital. But my major problems still persisted. I believe the reason I am here now is because God put my friend Rick back in my life after being apart for a few years. He brought me some information on noni and a bottle of noni juice, which gave me hope to go on. Within days of taking the noni juice, I started feeling better from problems that I had taken as a given in my life. The pain started leaving my body the first week very rapidly, and my skin went from a gray tone to a healthy glow. Most importantly, my spirit was back and I was able to see life for not for what I had lost but for what I didn't lose—my son and my friends. I will always be so humbly grateful to everyone who had brought forth the message of noni, providing me with this gift from God."

"I Was So Fatigued I Couldn't Do Anything"

James describes how noni helped him regain good health:

"I've been in the grocery industry for 29 years and was ready to own my own store. I was earning excellent money with great benefits and working 60 plus hours a week. That year I decided to get a flu shot. I had never had one before, but after receiving the flu shot my health really took a horrible turn. This is what I had to deal with on a daily basis: flu-like symptoms, swollen lymph nodes, sore throat, aching joints, headaches, rapid heart beat (resting heart rate was 100 beats per minute), short term memory loss, high cholesterol and triglycerides, high white blood count, low red blood count, pain from a swollen spleen and liver, pain in the right groin area, painfully swollen testes (with a lump in right one), blurred vision, mononucleosis, a positive testing for Epstein-Barr virus, and severe rashes on my face that wept and burned. In addition, I was so fatigued I couldn't do anything. And in a matter of just a few months I went from 225 pounds to 160 pounds. (I am well over six feet tall, so that was quite a dramatic and unwanted change.)

"In an attempt to rectify my problems, I went to a lot of different doctors, but nobody could give me anything that helped. In fact, a lot of the medicines made me feel even worse. I went to a physician out of town and had an endoscopy done. Nothing wrong could be identified. I also had a colonoscopy done. They found polyps—one large and precancerous—and removed all of them. I go back every two years and have more removed, and so far these have all been benign.

"After what seemed like an eternity, I still had no answers as to what was causing my problems. I went on my own to a dermatologist. He said I was having an allergic reaction to something. He scheduled tests to see if we could find what they were. The rashes just went away, so I didn't go back for the tests. A couple of months later the rashes came back, so I scheduled with the dermatologist again. When I got there I couldn't see the original doctor, so I saw a new doctor who had just arrived from the Mayo Clinic. He took one look at me and said I had poisons coming out of my body through my skin. He asked me to wait one minute and left the room. He came back fifteen minutes later, and said it wasn't poison, but that I was having an allergic reaction to something. I didn't like the two different versions, so I didn't go back.

"I went to another doctor and asked if my swollen spleen was causing some of my problems. He said, 'Well, when the spleen gets big enough, we'll take it out.' I asked him if this would help me feel better and he said that he didn't know the answer. Thus, I have not removed my spleen.

"I had a local doctor refer me to the Mayo Clinic to see if they could help me. After five days of testing, they could not come up with answers to what was causing my problems. They said all the symptoms were related to chronic fatigue syndrome. They had no tests for that or any medication to cure it. All they could do was schedule me to come back for three more days in the pain clinic. I decided not to do that because I simply wanted to find a way to get rid of the problems I was having.

"I went to another dermatologist to see if he could help with the recurring rashes. I told him my story. He was very fascinated. He felt I needed to have a blood work up for chemical and environmental poisoning. The results came back very high in most of the things he had me tested for. He recommended a doctor in Texas that specialized in this area. He recommended treatments of more blood tests and to go to Texas to live in a sterile environment to rid my body of these chemicals. My insurance company wasn't paying any of these bills, and I didn't have any money to do this, so I didn't go. The dermatologist said if I couldn't go, we should at least try to boost my immune system with vitamin supplements.

"However, I was already doing that. I had just joined a company that had non-caustic, environmentally safe, natural products to rid our home of the toxic chemicals we had been using. They also had great natural vitamins and other supplements. Because of this, I did see some improvement that let me work 30 to 40 hours per week on light duty.

"As if things weren't bad enough already, I fell and injured my neck and back. I damaged a lot of muscle tissue, suffered a slipped disc, developed bone spurs, a degenerative disc, and experienced the onset of severe arthritis in my neck and back. I have been off work for the

last year. In that time I was feeling pretty good, and had no rash outbreaks during that time. Then two months ago the rashes came back,
and all the old symptoms came back that I've had for the last six years.
I was devastated! I didn't know whether the work environment was the
original cause of the ailment, but being free of these symptoms for
almost a year showed me that environmental problems greatly exacerbated the problems I was having.

"About three months ago, my friend came over and told me about a
product called Tahitian Noni Juice™. We discussed trying it to see if
it would give me any relief from my multitude of problems. I was so
excited about trying this product that I bought a bottle from her and
began taking it that night. What a taste!

"After being on noni juice for only 5 days I began to see fantastic
results! Here are some:

- I had four teeth that hurt clear down to the jawbone. I had x-rays
  taken and nothing showed up. I'm totally pain free now!
- I haven't been able to breath out of my right nostril ever since I can
  remember. I am able to breath out of it now!
- I've had chronic pain in both knees since junior high. I have no pain
  in my knees now!
- For the last two months I have had trouble focusing my eyes, so I
  could not read first thing in the morning. I have no problems now!

"After taking noni for 10 days, I sleep through the night, contrary to
what was happening for the previous two or three months. After about
two weeks on noni, my right toes, which have hurt since having toe
surgery a year ago, now have no pain!

"After about three weeks on noni, I noticed a big reduction in my
constant fatigue. I have more energy than I've had in six years. I no
longer have to take naps just to make it through the day.

"After five weeks, I could honestly say that the pain in my testes and
my right groin area was almost completely gone. My neck and back
problem? I now have less pain and more mobility, so I feel it is also
helping the injury and the arthritis that I had in those areas.

"I have now decreased my dosage of noni from 8 to 6 tablespoons, twice a day. Though things aren't perfect, I have seen some dramatic improvements in my health, all of which were a result of this miracle fruit!"

"She Was Almost a Skeleton"

Marvin and Betsy give a moving account of how noni helped their infant granddaughter recover from a serious illness:

"We have a 17-month-old granddaughter, Carrie, who has been very sick since she was 5 months old. She has been on an oxygen machine for a year. She has had numerous tests completed, all of which revealed nothing. She weighed just over ten pounds when born, yet at 17 months, she was almost a skeleton. During this time, she had never been strong enough to walk.

"Because of Carrie's problems, especially with breathing, her doctors prescribed asthma treatments of albuteral three times a day just to ease her breathing. In July her parents brought her to Utah for five weeks and spent a lot of time at the hospital where she had surgery for reflux problems. They were not given any encouragement on getting Carrie off the oxygen. They took her to the National Jewish Hospital in Denver, Colorado (which is one of the top respiratory hospitals in the country) where they consulted with the hospital's top doctor. He felt she had contracted a virus at 5 months that had permanently scarred her lungs and airways. The air sacs in the bottom of her lungs were collapsed and were retaining fluid. The doctor told them if they were lucky by the time Carrie was 8 or 10 years old her airways might grow large enough for her to be able to breathe on her own.

"In October we heard a woman say she had been on oxygen for two years and had been able to get off of it because of noni. So, we sent a bottle to Carrie's parents. Her mom was reluctant as Carrie was on seven medications, including prednisone. With coaxing she gave her a spoonful twice a day in her bottle. After two weeks we got a message on our answering machine that said, "Daddy your noni juice is magic! Carrie's respirator specialist cut her oxygen by 25 percent today!" One week later we got another call. "Daddy it isn't magic, it's a miracle!"

We cut Carrie's oxygen another 25 percent. By the fifth week on noni she got off all her medication along with a further reduction in need for oxygen.

"Carrie is now gaining weight at a normal level. For the first time in a year she can fight a cold without antibiotics. Her energy levels are dramatically higher than they were before she started on noni. She has started walking, and we have high hopes it won't be long until Carrie can play like other children, without being tied to an oxygen machine."

"I Have Been to Countless Doctors"

Bill Tramel details his account involving noni's role in helping him regain his health after a lifetime of accidents and health conditions:

"My lifetime of accidents began in 1950 when I was eleven years old. My pony threw me when he accidentally stepped on a snake, and I suffered a compound fracture of the wrist. In 1957 I broke my left knee in a toboggan accident and wore a cast for four months. In 1963 my hand went through a double V-belt pulley, cutting off my right index finger and crushing all other joints of the fingers on my right hand. I had an infection in my joints for several months.

"In 1979 I was in a motorcycle accident and fractured my back in two places and dislocated my neck. Twenty-five percent of one vertebra was shattered and one third of the other vertebra broke off, slid to the side, and healed crooked. Also several discs had ruptured. As a result of that accident I spent 30 days in the hospital, wore a neck and back brace for three months, and couldn't work for one and a half years. To top it all off, in 1985 I slipped off the top of an auto transport semi and experienced severe back and neck injuries. Consequently, my working days were over, and I could no longer do physical work of any kind.

"Since 1979 I have been to countless doctors, chiropractors, therapists, etc., trying to get relief from the pain due to rheumatoid arthritis. I took sleep medications, anti-inflammatory medications, pain medications, and high blood pressure pills, all of which had to be increased periodically. As a result of all my problems, I suffered from depression.

"In August of 1996, I had an MRI which showed the bottom of my spine had suffered extensive deterioration. At this time I had severe pain in both of my legs as well as my lower back. Not surprisingly, my doctor was not optimistic about my ever leading a normal or pain-free life again.

"A couple of months later, I was introduced to something called Tahitian Noni Juice™. I started taking two ounces per day. In 30 days noni juice normalized my blood pressure, and even after I had it rechecked several times, it continued to stay normal. At that time I also quit taking my anti-inflammatory medication, and in about two months I could for the first time in five years walk up and down steps without any pain. Soon after that the pain in my right knee started subsiding, and after about three weeks I could drive without experiencing much pain in my legs.

"It is the first time since 1979, when I broke my back, that I am drug free, and I thank noni that my pain, fatigue, and swelling have all either disappeared or become minimal."

"She Would Not Live Out the Day"

Roger K. provides this incredible account concerning his mother's comeback from the brink of death using noni juice:

"I became familiar with noni in February and proceeded to hear all of the stories about wonderful things that noni juice was doing. That was very interesting to me, but until you have the opportunity to experience first hand noni juice results, all of the testimonials are a little removed from you. My mother, who was 92 years old, has been in a nursing home for the past five years. Last August, while in the nursing home, she became dehydrated to the point that she lapsed into a coma and her doctor called me to say that she would not live out the day.

"Contrary to the doctor's warning, my mother did pull out of the coma; however, she was left in a vegetative state. She had no vision, no hearing, and spoke only a couple of times since August. Typical nursing home scenario—tipped back in a chair, mouth and eyes open, and totally unresponsive. At Christmas, I visited her for six days and had the total response of 5 words. I really doubt that she was aware of who I was. Two weeks ago I decided to put noni to the test. I sent two bottles to the nursing home and asked the head nurse, Linda, to give her one ounce in the morning and one ounce in the evening. Linda laughed and said, 'Oh well, the juice can't hurt her.'

"Yesterday Linda called me to update the results of noni juice and Mom. She is now sitting up, can now see, and is talking to all of the nurses and is very alert. Linda's comment was, 'You are in for a big surprise when you come to visit again.' If you ever wanted to see a 58-year-old man have tears of joy, yesterday was it. Noni works! This story is unbelievable but true for someone that had been given up on by her doctor. He has now started to get interested in noni juice. This juice is truly a gift from God.

"P.S. Linda (the nurse) has now started to take noni juice."

"My Father Prayed to God That My Life Be Spared"

Gloria Schanely relates how noni helped her achieve an incredible recovery from various health conditions:

"My story is a remarkable one because it started many years ago, at the age of five, and now I am 44 years old! I am a mother of three beautiful daughters, and three gorgeous grandbabies. I am an Official Court Interpreter for the Spanish related cases in Central Florida, and have been for the past 10 years. I have also been a radio and TV broadcaster for the past 18 years, a soloist and upcoming short story book author, too. Since I can remember, I have suffered from different ailments, including constipation, sinusitis, PMS (I call it pre-, present and post-menstrual syndrome), gastritis, depression, arthritis, the aftermath of meningitis, migraines, and weight problems (I'm 40 pounds overweight). At the age of five, I remember my mother sitting me on the toilet for hours, due to severe constipation. Sometimes it would take me two or three days in a row to empty my bowels. At the age of 16 I tried to take my life, and swallowed half a bottle of Dristan (about 16-20 pills) because I would go into these terrible depressions. I have always noticed I have been a nervous kind of person, but in a good way. I have always been a positive thinking person and work very hard and put in very long hours at what I do. But a terrible and violent marriage that ended in 1986 really brought stress into my life and clouded my thinking.

"Even though I am a committed Christian and come from a good family where both my parents were ministers in a church, I felt a real emptiness. This emptiness, combined with chemical imbalances, would send me into terrible depressions and mood swings. I went out one evening in 1985 (going through the worst part of my separation) and had a few drinks. As a result, I got into a car accident that affected my left hip, my left leg, and my left foot and big toe. Later, arthritis started developing in these areas. The pain started intensifying as years progressed, until I moved to Florida in 1990, and went to the doctor. As conditions worsened, I had to lift my left leg with my left hand to get into my car because it did not bend up or lift up by itself. Then in 1986, after my divorce, I developed gastritis, and it became so bad that as of last year (1998), I had to take prescription Tagamet 3 three times a day. There were a number of foods I was not able to digest, like tomatoes, pizza, beans, or bean soups, and needless to say, even milk was out of the picture!

"Often enough, there were nights I would wake up at 2 or 3 in the morning with pain, and have to run to the store for medication because I would run out of the prescription medicine. I was eating 6 or 7 meals a day, just to take the pain away, as the intake of food takes away the burning sensation of gastritis.

"In addition to these problems, I had also developed acute sinusitis and there was not a morning that I would not wake up and be totally congested, having to gargle, wash out my nose and sinuses with salty water, and continually spit. Finally, to top everything off, in April 1997, due to an infected mosquito bite, I contracted viral meningitis. I was hospitalized immediately, and between life and death that night, my father prayed to God that my life be spared.

"Thanks to my father's prayers, I was spared. However, for the next three months I could not think right, walk well, or drive. My vision was almost as if it were in fast-forward motion. I lost most of my contracted jobs with the court, and I lost my live radio show which I had hosted for the last three years. I still was not functioning right for two years after this, and started developing intense headaches and migraines. This continued up through March of 1999.

"In December of 1998, I was driving on my way to work when my mind went blank. I was suffering a panic attack, where I didn't know who I was, what I was doing driving down this road, what day it was, or anything! It was the scariest thing I had experienced, and I broke down and cried. I ended up just sitting there praying until I recovered and drove back home and slept for five hours.

"After this, I became very depressed and kept thinking to myself that I had definitely come to the end of life with my mind going down the drain, waking up every morning with a different source of pain! If it wasn't my sinus, it was my arthritis. If it wasn't my gastritis, it was another migraine. And if it happened to be the first day of my menstrual period, I would not be able to go to work or even get up! After giving birth to my second daughter (22 years ago), I had terrible PMS every single month of my life. The clotting was terrible and it felt sometimes like birth pains when the clots would clear the uterus and were discharged.

"In January of 1999, I was contacted via the internet by a man that I now consider a God-sent angel, who told me some pretty fascinating stories that tickled my brain. These stories were from other people that had recovered from migraines, gastritis, arthritis, cancer, high blood pressure and many more disorders. I decided to drive two hours to the coast and meet him. I bought two bottles of noni juice and gave one to my dad and mom, and another one for a friend, but I didn't start taking it until February because I was too skeptical. But I finally relented.

"To start, my dose was one ounce of noni juice in the morning and one ounce at night. After the first bottle though, I still needed improvement, so I decided to take another ounce in the afternoon.

"After about six weeks I woke up that morning without pain, which was the first time in years. Thank you, Jesus!

"And it didn't stop there. My pain has literally disappeared! When I have felt a migraine approaching, I just take another ounce. Last month, I went to the beach the very first day of my period, which I hadn't been able to do in years. I didn't even detect the customary menstrual odor that comes with it, nor was the clotting so severe. My sinus condition has totally cleared up, and I don't wake up congested in the morning. I am sleeping like a baby, and I don't wake up with gastritis pains any more. Last week, I was once again able to start eating tomatoes and other foods that I previously had to steer clear of. I have placed all my Tagamet 3 prescriptions, Advil, Tylenol 3, Motrin, and Excedrin Migraine up on my kitchen shelf away from sight.

"The most remarkable thing though, is that I am now able to think straight. I have my confidence back, and I feel that my brain is balanced. And as far as my work goes, I have the 'edge' necessary to get the job done. In essence, my energy has been renewed and I don't feel 'brain dead.' Even my friends at work have to tell me to slow down because I am typing too fast for them! I feel happy, satisfied, content, and ready to help anyone else find the miracle I discovered in noni juice!"

"Every Move I Made Resulted In Total Pain"

Toni, portions of whose story we have already reviewed, details her successful battle with chronic fatigue, arthritis and other conditions using noni:

"I am a 54-year-old grandmother of nine, with a body that was slowly falling apart. Because of being overweight for such a long time, I was making myself ill. Because of my arthritis there were days when every move I made my body reacted with total pain. The cartilage was gone in both of my knees, eaten up by the arthritis. In May of 1996 I had a total replacement surgery on my right knee. For years I took arthritis medicine, all of which made me sick. So about a year ago I stopped taking the medicine.

"While I was in the hospital my diabetes went out of control. I took shots while in the hospital and four pills a day after returning home. Now, after being on Tahitian Noni Juice™ juice for three and a half months, my blood-sugar reading regularly registers at 78. I also have CFS (chronic fatigue syndrome), high blood pressure, bladder infections, respiratory problems, asthma, seizure disorder, and sleep apnea, just to name a few. I was on pills of all kinds and not sleeping at night, so I also took nerve pills to help me get to sleep.

"In July I was visiting my family in Indiana. My sister and mom started telling me I should try a particular new product called noni, and about how much better they were feeling. I was there for several days and in a lot of pain. That's when I gave in, and my life has made a complete turn around ever since. It didn't happen over night, since there were so many things wrong with me.

"I was seeing my family doctor because of a car accident on August 28, 1996. He hadn't seen me for a few months and could see quite a difference immediately. All the tests he ran were much improved. Blood pressure, skin color, chest and bruising from the accident healed much faster. He was very interested in seeing what noni would do for my CFS. I told him how I was not tired all the time and that I could actually walk across the room. Today I am not taking anything for pain, or using my cane to walk. I am also able to keep up with all of my grandchildren who live close by and are in and out all the time.

"As a bonus I have lost 20 pounds for the first time in 30 years. The weight loss itself will help everything wrong with me. I feel better, have more energy, am less stressed and am sleeping better at night. I am a much nicer person to be around. I am a true believer in noni."

"The Cancer Was In Complete Remission"

Angela, 49 years old, provides the details of her fantastic recovery from a near-fatal bout with brain cancer:

"In April 1997 I lost the use of the left side of my body. The doctors couldn't figure out what was wrong so they put a soft boot on my left leg up to my knee so that I could walk. A few weeks later after a sauna at the gym, I had a seizure. I was taken to the hospital and x-rays showed that I had a brain tumor, which had caused my brain to swell, resulting in the seizure. They said it was an anaplastic oligodendroglioma, which is a very rare type of cancer with an extremely low survival rate. Immediately a neurosurgeon operated on me, but he could not remove the entire tumor without affecting vitally functioning parts of my brain. I was then given six weeks of radiation and one year of chemotherapy.

"Not surprisingly, the chemotherapy made me deathly ill with weakness, nausea, vomiting and fever. I lost 35 pounds. During the next few months, I was in and out of the hospital and was too weak to participate in any of my normal activities. I had to take early retirement from work and was put on permanent long-term disability. My oncologist told me that I was terminal, that there was no hope. Despite this, I firmly decided that I was going to live.

"A short time later, I started taking about eight ounces of Tahitian Noni Juice™ a day on the advice of a friend. After calling the office of a nutritionist familiar with using noni for cancer, I increased my consumption to a full bottle a day for the next four weeks. Next I went to Texas to consult with a nutritionist and homeopathic practitioner. His tests indicated that I had the body of a 73-year-old, though I was 48. Based on the results of his tests he added various supplements and advised me to continue drinking eight ounces of noni juice daily.

"Several days into my treatment, I noticed my strength returning and I started to gain weight. I spent the next year working on healing myself. I used meditation, visualization, hands-on healing, and motivational tapes and books. I modified my diet to include more fruits and vegetables and tried to eliminate pesticides and preservatives by eating organic foods. As I gained strength I started an organic garden, revamped my backyard, joined a bowling league, and took golf lessons. For about eight months, I drank about eight ounces of noni juice daily.

"In April 1999, my doctors told me the cancer was in complete remission. Though the left side of my body has still not regained complete functionality, I can now live a comparatively normal life. Since then I have been taking a multiple vitamin/mineral supplement and drinking four ounces of noni juice a day. In late August, I plan to spend six weeks touring California, going on a cruise to Alaska, and visiting Las Vegas. I am extremely thankful that I was able to find a natural way to beat cancer. And thanks to noni, I now have my life back again!"

The Noni Phenomenon: What the Experts Think

PREVIOUS CHAPTERS OF this book have provided a comprehensive review of scientific, anecdotal and case study material concerning the wonderful health benefits of noni. However, one of the richest sources of feedback that I received in my survey concerning noni use comes from the 50 doctors and health professionals who both use noni and recommend it to their patients, as well as other individuals who have an in-depth knowledge of noni's powerful life-changing capabilities. This chapter provides a balanced mixture of expert opinions and commentary centering around noni and its value for today's health world.

Floyd Holdman

Floyd Holdman was one of the first individuals to become heavily involved in the marketing and distribution of noni in the United States.

"For over 25 years I have traveled as a photographer to over 52 countries around the world. My clients have included National Geographic, General Mills, Sony, RCA and many, many others.

"My favorite place in the entire world to visit and photograph is Tahiti. The pristine environment combined with the beauty and friendliness of the people make it a literal paradise on earth. The colorful flowers on the trees and shrubs are echoed in the crystal clear waters by the myriad of colorful fish. The lush greenery of the islands is rivaled only by the turquoise green of the lagoons.

"In the midst of all this, grows a miracle fruit called *noni* (or *nono* by the native Tahitians). I was first introduced to this peculiar fruit in 1996. After six weeks of drinking about an once of noni juice a day, I noticed that the arthritic pain in my hands was gone. I began to share this new-found discovery with many of my friends and family members. To my and their amazement, many of them found relief from some very serious health challenges, as well as experienced an overall improvement in their well-being.

"Noni is a miracle from paradise that the whole world needs to hear about."

Dr. Ralph Heinicke

The following is an excerpt from interview questions presented to Dr. Ralph Heinicke, considered by many to be the foremost pioneer in noni research.

Q: *Tell us about how you became involved with noni. What sparked your interest in it?*

A: After I obtained my Ph.D. in 1950, I went to work for the Pineapple Research Institute in Hawaii. At that time the Institute had a wonderful Hawaiian research worker, Carl Farden. He was descended from members of the royal Hawaiian families on his mother's side and his wife was one of the few remaining full-blooded members of the Hawaiian royal family. Carl was proud of his Hawaiian heritage and graciously shared with us newcomers to the Islands tales about old Hawaii. From him and his well-placed Hawaiian friends we learned the male Hawaiian hula dance, the locations of the old heiaus on Oahu, and the various Hawaiian plants that the kahunas used to cure the health problems of their patients. Noni was one of the most important of these remedies.

Although my officially assigned task was to isolate the protease bromelain from the pineapple fruit, as a hobby I investigated the milk clotting activity of all of the local Hawaiian plants. To my surprise I found that noni juice contained from twenty to thirty times as much milk clotting activity (a reputed measure of protease activity) as did pineapple fruit juice. Thus my first interest in noni was as a possible competitor of bromelain.

Several years later, after I had transferred to the company that would become Dole, the primary market for bromelain was the pharmaceutical market. Herb Cornuelle, the president of Dole, asked me whether I could assure him that a better plant or microbial product would not supplant bromelain in the pharmaceutical market. I assured him that a better product certainly would be made and that I hoped that our department would make it.

As a result of this commitment, I carefully monitored the progress of all potential competitors. Only three products appeared to be potential competitors at that time, noni fruit, DMSO and a synthetic drug called Dilantin®. All these products had extensive histories of medical applications. The reported physiological results were all similar to those that the drug companies had found for bromelain.

At that time (1956) I did not believe that noni was a serious commercial competitor for bromelain. Dole had several thousand acres of closely planted pineapple plants that could be harvested mechanically. The island of Oahu had only several hundred scattered noni trees. The fruit would have had to be hand harvested. Even though noni juice was as good a source of product as pineapple stem juice, the costs of the juice would have been prohibitive for a commercial venture.

Q: After hearing the claims about what noni could do, were you ever skeptical?

A: At no time did I doubt the claims made for noni juice. I had several reasons for this belief. I had seen the data that various drug companies had developed on the pharmaceutical efficacy of bromelain. (These data came from the time when the pharmacological potency of commercial bromelain was still high.)

What few people realize is that no other plant product has ever undergone such an intensive and extensive pharmaceutical investigation as bromelain. Pharmaceutical companies generally only publish work that is pertinent to their pending commercial products. Therefore, much of the work on bromelain was never published.

One drug company in particular, the one that believed that the discovery of the medical uses of bromelain was one of the major medical discoveries in recent times, tested the use of bromelain alone and in combination with other drugs to treat almost every known ailment. Their data showed success in treating such problems as some types of cancer, some types of arthritis, some types of emphysema, some types of senility, some types of intractable infections, some types of diabetes, some types of blood pressure problems—the list went on and on. Therefore I was not at all surprised to hear that drinking noni juice cured some of these same problems. I knew that good quality bromelain and noni juice contained the same active pharmaceutical ingredient. Therefore, the almost miraculous results reported for noni were exactly what I had expected.

Q: *What pushed you to pursue your investigation of noni?*
A: When a group of local entrepreneurs in Hawaii began considering the possibility of producing a noni-based health drink, they asked me to join them and to develop and provide the technical information. By this time I had already developed the xeronine-system concept. I also knew that bromelain and "nonain" (the "protease" mixture from noni fruit) were similar plant sulfhydryl enzymes and that both owed their effectiveness as health-promoting products to some substance other than the protease. I believed that I could show that noni contained the same xeronine-system that I had discovered in the pineapple plant.

I should mention that the xeronine-system occurs in all plants, animals and in most—but definitely not all— microorganisms. However, only a few plants have sufficient amounts of the xeronine-system for these plants to be a dietary source of this system. Noni fruit juice is one of the best known available sources of this system.

Q: *What has been the most fulfilling aspect of your work and experience with noni?*
A: As have many other people, I have always been interested in the health promoting aspects of certain foods that are highly esteemed by certain cultures. When the early American explorer, Ponce de Leone, came to America searching for the fountain of youth, he stopped in Cuba before going on to Florida.

When I came to Hawaii and began studying some of the health promoting aspects of the pineapple plant, I thought that Ponce de Leone had made a mistake by not staying in Cuba. Cuba had excellent pineapple. Drinking pineapple juice was as close as he could have gotten to finding the fountain of youth. (At that time the island that was to become Cuba did not have any noni trees.)

In 1958 we had experimental data that, if properly applied and promoted, could have alleviated much of our country's problems with high cholesterol and high blood pressure. Our data showed that the problem was not high cholesterol in our diet but a faulty cholesterol regulatory synthesizing system in our bodies. This belief is now being accepted today.

Thus, for many decades we had an empirical cure. We had the experimental data, both on animals and on people, to prove that the proposed program worked, but at the time that we did the research, we did not know why the system worked. Also, because of conflicts with the advertising program and internal maneuvering within the company for position, Dole decided that they would discontinue the health research aspects of the program and use a more conventional technique to sell pineapple products. For this reason our cholesterol research, which we had carried out with Dr. Ross of the University of Hawaii and the medical group, was never made available to the public.

A few years after I had left Dole I developed the xeronine-system concept. Now I knew the nature of the unknown physiologically active ingredient that occurred in noni and in the Hawaiian pineapple. However, now that I had the answer, I no longer had a vehicle for getting the story to the public and I no longer had access to a fruit that was an acceptable source of the xeronine-system. Having an answer to critical and expensive health problems but not being able to get the story or a suitable product to the public frustrated me.

Little did I dream that there would be such a successful answer to my problems. When Kerry and Kim Asay contacted me and told me that they, along with John Wadsworth and Stephen Story, had developed a noni product that could be immediately made available to the people and that they could spread the story, I was practically incredulous. This is what I had dreamed of. But I do not believe in dreams.

Without question, this was the most satisfying experience that I have had working with noni. It was something that I had hoped might happen. It is something that I know this world needed.

Q: What do you think the future holds for noni?
A: The future for the xeronine-system and noni is unbelievably exciting. At present we know that merely drinking noni juice regularly has brought relief to many people who have had serious health problems. Many of these problems had not responded to traditional pharmaceutical treatments. However, today we are just beginning to explore what xeronine does at the molecular level, where it adsorbs onto a receptor protein, what it does when it is in position, and how this affects the hormones that might adsorb onto an adjacent site on the same receptor protein. When we have this information, doctors will be able to treat our health problems more effectively.

I believe that the xeronine-system concepts will split into two separate but complementary approaches. In one approach, developed by the pharmaceutical industry and administered by doctors, the companies will concentrate on working with pure compounds. This will enable the doctor to deliver specific amounts of components to specific organs. The health organizations need this approach to deal with certain severe health problems, such as treating third degree burns or treating diseased organs, or injecting components of the system into areas close to joint replacements.

The other approach, which is the current approach, will deal with nutrition. This is where the market for noni can expand greatly as people realize the importance of supplying the body with an external source of the xeronine system.

I believe that under ideal conditions the body can make xeronine without requiring pre-formed components from the diet. I also strongly believe that with our modern diet and our modern lifestyle the majority of us are seriously deficient in components of the xeronine-system. Stress, growth, tissue repair and environmental poisons all increase our need for more xeronine while at the same time decreasing the body's innate ability for synthesizing the components of the system.

At present most people who are taking noni take it once a day. Yet I know of many people who eat food three or four times a day. Noni is a food; it is not a drug. It is a unique food that is exceptionally rich in the components for a critical building block that our body constantly requires. In the future we may discover new schedules for taking noni that will increase the effectiveness of noni for certain health problems. We may also find that combining noni with certain foods may have a synergistic effect. These are all exciting areas for increasing the effectiveness of an already very effective product.

The combination of the increased use of noni in the diet of the average American plus the availability of purified forms on the xeronine-system in time of a medical crisis bodes well for our future health. The proper use of noni in our diet can appreciably reduce the onset of health problems and the availability of the pure components of the xeronine-system can help treat many acute health problems.

Q: *How do you value the historical and cultural links between noni and the various island cultures?*

A: I have a great respect for the traditions of different cultures. Their traditions reflect centuries of experience of living together and of exploring their environment for treatments for health problems. Of course, those treatments that were successful were incorporated into their traditions.

Noni was one of the most important of the medicinal plants that the Tahitians discovered very early in their history. When they went exploring the ocean for new lands, noni was one of the plants that they carried with them. This is how noni came to Hawaii.

I also respect and attempt to understand some of their accessory suggestions and operations, such as picking certain plants "under the dark of the moon" or accompanying the administration of the medicine with dances and music. The "under the dark of the moon" probably is a reference to the average weather conditions that exist locally at a certain time of the month as measured by the phase of the moon. Picking a medicinal plant at the improper time can seriously affect the potential health promoting ingredients in the plant. (I have abundant data on the effect of weather on the pharmacological potency of the pineapple plant.)

The medicine men found through experience that the emotional state of the patient affected the efficacy of the medicine. Their dances around the patient were an important part of the treatment. Today a biochemist would say that the medicine men were using a two-component treatment; the noni supplied the xeronine and the dances stimulated the brain to release specific hormones. Both the xeronine and the hormone were necessary for certain protein receptors to become fully active.

In our modern culture, if we cannot find a convenient medicine man who can do a convincing ceremonial dance, we can put on a Mozart record and achieve the same effect—providing, of course, one likes Mozart.

Q: Please explain what you envisioned happening with your initial work with noni. Did you ever dream that it would evolve into what it has?

A: The old sage who said, "Build a better mouse trap, and the world will beat a path to your door" knew nothing about modern business.

I knew that noni juice had the potential for alleviating many critical health problems and that the world needed this juice. Furthermore, I knew that the physiologically active ingredients in both commercial bromelain and noni were the same. They were a group of molecules that I have called the xeronine-system since the end product of a series of reactions is the alkaloid xeronine. Because they were the same, the extensive database of information built up on the actions of commercial bromelain by drug companies and various research groups also applies to noni. This was a powerful story. Not only was no one beating a path to my door, but I was also having difficulty in finding the proper doors to beat on.

From my experiences at Dole, I knew that getting a chemical story to the public would be difficult, expensive and probably long in coming. Therefore when a group of local entrepreneurs established a small company to produce noni juice in Hawaii, they initially planned to sell the juice in Hawaii where a small local market for the juice existed. Then as its reputation became established, they planned to slowly expand to the mainland United States. Unfortunately, when we needed additional money, the bankers were not impressed with this plan and we never produced any noni product for sale.

When Kerry Asay called me about seven years later, he told me that he had a bottled noni product in a warehouse and that he could put together an organization that would be able to take the noni-story to the public. I was interested in what he was planning to do, but frankly, I was not overly optimistic; I had already been through one noni venture. Later when I visited Kerry and Kim Asay and met John Wadsworth and Stephen Story, I was impressed. I felt that if any group could produce and market noni juice, this was the group that would do it. I believed then that this group would be a successful operation that would do well in a niche market, providing a much-needed product to the people.

What this group has done with noni is what I had fantasized might happen. That this group was able to produce an eminently acceptable product in large volumes and to present the noni story to the public in such a short time is something that I did not believe was possible.

Q: What is your favorite story/testimony involving the use of noni?
A: When one thinks about some of the almost miraculous stories, such as the person with supposedly terminal emphysema getting out of the oxygen tent, going home and living a busy and happy life after she started taking noni, it is hard to pick out one particular story.

One story that particularly intrigued me was the story told by a 93-year-old woman who had been having hearing problems. This woman started by telling us that she did not believe in testimonials. However, she happened to have an interesting experience that she wanted to share with us. On her previous visit to the doctor he had given her a battery of sound perception tests. On her second visit he wanted to conduct a few more tests. As the doctor was proceeding with his tests, suddenly his assistant, who was operating the recording machine in the adjoining room, murmured a quiet, "Darn! I wiped out all of the data."

The lady turned to the doctor, who had barely heard this exclamation, and told him to tell his assistant not to worry about losing the previous data since it was no longer valid. She had been taking noni only after the first test. Her hearing was now fine. Many of us who had the pleasure of talking with her can agree that her hearing was excellent.

Q: *Why do you think noni is destined to become a household name?*
A: Only a few years ago, not many Americans had heard of St. John's wort. Now, hundreds of thousands take it on a daily basis. Noni is currently in a similar situation. That will change soon as more doctors compare the action of these two plants, as well as that of other natural and pharmaceutical products. Noni is truly in a class by itself. Noni frequently alleviates problems that conventional pharmaceutical drugs have failed to cure. Furthermore, it does this without causing damaging side effects. This is a story that the newspapers and the media are not adequately presenting.

When the breakthrough finally comes—and it will—then noni will become a household term very quickly.

Q: *How do you use noni products? And your family and friends?*
A: Being a scientist and not having animals that I can use for experiments, I frequently investigate different effects of noni on myself. (Since I know my name, address, blood pressure, telephone number, marital status, weight and age, any observations that I make can be considered as scientific data and not anecdotal reports.)

After having lived for thirty years in Hawaii and having gone swimming and sailing at every opportunity without using suntan lotion, hats, shirts or sunglasses, I am now paying for these indiscretions. Some of my skin cancers can be easily and quickly removed by burning. Some are so deep that they can only be treated by a special operation. This operation is like mining for gold except the object is to keep on mining until the lode (cancer cells) runs out. Each minute shovelful of cells is analyzed for cancer cells. Since this operation has the potential for being bloody, this gave me an excellent opportunity to conduct a test of the effect of noni on thinning the blood.

People who have "thick" blood frequently benefit from taking noni, which helps bring the viscosity of the blood back to normal. What I was interested in finding out was how taking large amounts of noni before an operation would affect the blood. Would it thin it effectively, or could it even thin it too much?

The day before the operation I took a teaspoon of noni every two hours throughout the day. The morning of the start of the operation I took two tablespoons full of noni. Since I did not want to worry the doctor, I did not tell him what I had done. I knew that if my blood were too thin, the worst that would happen would be that the doctor would have a messy time and I would have a badly bruised face.

During the operation I casually asked the doctor how things were going. He said things were excellent. I then specifically asked him about my bleeding. He assured me that he was having no trouble with bleeding. When the operation was finally finished (six hours later) and the incision was closed, he told me that since the operation was close to the eyes that I would have the worst case of black and swollen eyes that I'd ever had. He told me not to worry; however, he also warned me not to go out because I would scare people. He then gave me a prescription for a painkiller.

I told him that I did not believe that I would have black eyes and that I would not need a painkiller. Of course he did not believe me, since he had performed that operation many times. As soon as I got home, I immediately started taking noni every two hours. Frankly, I did not look so good when I got home. However, after four hours, all of the swelling had gone down and I had no black eyes. In fact, the change was so dramatic that we took a picture to show to the doctor. The next morning my eyes were again swollen, but still with no black or blue discoloration. (I had not set the alarm clock to take noni every two hours during the night.) Again I started taking noni every two hours. Within a couple hours, the swelling had disappeared. However, if I delayed taking the noni every two hours, the swelling began to reappear. Thus for an acute injury, which such an operation truly is, one should take noni frequently. For this particular operation, every two hours was a satisfactory scheduling.

At no time during the day or night was I bothered by pain. Of course, I had known about this aspect of noni for years, so I was not surprised. When the doctor saw me two days after the operation, he was surprised at how rapidly the wound had healed. He said that even with young patients, he rarely had incisions heal so rapidly.

Six months later I had another similar operation on a different part of my face. Again the results were the same—minimal swelling, no black and blue discoloration, no pain and rapid healing.

I had another interesting experience concerning the effect of noni on healing. (Once again, since I have all of the vital statistics, I feel justified in considering this scientific data rather than an anecdote.) This time the healing was of bone tissue.

While in Honolulu, a root canal surgeon failed to find one of the three nerves that he was attempting to remove from the roots of one of my teeth. In a blind attempt to find the nerve, he kept drilling. In fact he drilled through the tooth into the tissue. He then filled the tooth cavity and the hole that he made in the tissue with silver amalgam! By the time we moved to Louisville, an abscess had developed on this root since the old nerve was still in the root canal. Since the abscess appeared to be draining well, the dentist suggested waiting a while. However, two days before I left for Utah, I had real trouble with the abscess. When I returned, I located a first class root canal specialist. He located and removed the hidden root nerve and disconnected the silver amalgam from the root canal. Because of erosion of the jawbone by the abscess, he told me to return within a year and that he would then repair the jawbone.

After a year (of course, I was regularly taking noni the entire time) I returned and had a new x-ray taken of the tooth and jaw. When he saw the x-ray, he shook his head in disbelief. He told me that the x-ray showed what theoretically should have happened but unfortunately rarely does. The bone had completely regenerated. There was no need for him to do anything. This experience convinced him that noni had real merit in promoting the healing of tissues and even of bone tissue.

Noni has greatly helped my daughter-in-law. (Since I do not know her weight or her pulse rate, I shall have to classify this report as anecdotal.) Last year she developed severe arthritis in her knee joints. This was so severe that she frequently used a cane for walking. She went to the best rheumatologist for help. The standard arthritis drugs gave her no relief. Even carefully spaced cortisone injections gave her only temporary relief. Finally she tried noni. The next day she did a little dance for me. As long as she takes noni, she has no problem with arthritis.

Anne Hirazumi, Ph.D.

Dr. Hirazumi has provided the world with some of the most recent and pertinent research regarding noni's ability to strengthen the immune system and fight various health conditions, most notably cancer. Today she is considered one of the premiere researchers of noni.

"My experience with noni had what you could call a 'nonglamorous' beginning. Ten years ago I had a dog named Brownie who was very sick. Of course, I really wanted to do something to help him regain his health. My father suggested that I give him some noni juice. I had never heard of any such thing as 'noni juice' before that. Telling my father this, he explained that it had been noni juice that helped his friend experience marvelous results in his recovery from cancer.

"Intrigued, I gave some noni juice to Brownie, at first putting it in his water bowl. He wouldn't touch it. But then I put my hand in his bowl, and he drank it from my hand. Soon, he was drinking more of the water/noni combination than what he previously drank of just water.

"Before I knew it, Brownie started getting better. I was really shocked. He started running around, he regained his appetite, and he just started looking like his old self again. All I could think was, "Wow!—the noni juice really helped him." It was this experience that inspired me to become a graduate student in pharmacology at the University of Hawaii so that I could study the biological effects of noni juice."

Kelly Olsen

Kelly is Vice President of Sales and Marketing for Morinda, Inc., located in Provo, Utah. He has been instrumental in bringing noni to North America and the rest of the world.

"When thinking about how noni has affected my life, it is something that I could write about for hours. I think the things that I feel so strongly about noni happen at several levels.

"At the most fundamental level is it's comprehensive ability to effect a positive benefit in the human body. It continually amazes me as I hear the testimonials from our consumers. They are far reaching, comprehensive, and sometimes even miraculous. I know there are nay-sayers out there and people who blithely attribute these health recoveries to the placebo effect or maybe mere coincidence, but I've looked in their eyes and talked with them. These aren't imagined benefits. Noni changes people.

"In order to be effective, noni must be processed correctly, the ingredients must be protected, and the formula and fulfillment must be correct. Individuals that jump on the bandwagon with a product sourced from broker 'X' with their nifty new label trivialize the product, the history and the potential of noni.

"Noni represents hope on another significant level. We have partnered up with those who know noni best—the people. They pick it, transport it, and process it for us. Many of them are also the ones who are benefitting financially from this movement. It is like we are involved with something that demands very special attention beyond those of simple manufacturing methods. I believe it is a special gift from God."

Dr. Gary Tran

The following provides excerpts from interview questions presented to Dr. Gary Tran, a veterinarian who has used noni to successfully treat thousands of animals for various health conditions.

Q: *Explain how you became involved with noni. What sparked your interest in it?*

A: I first heard about noni juice when a friend living in Irvine, California, sent me the literature about noni juice, including some promotional writings and a half dozen scientific reprints of noni research around the world.

Q: *After hearing the claims about what noni could do, were you ever skeptical?*

A: As a veterinarian practicing holistic veterinary medicine, I have been bombarded by promotional literature making all kinds of claims, substantiated and non-substantiated all the time. But most of these claims were not backed by genuine research. At least noni has some basic research proving that it was anticarcinogenic, analgesic, and anti-retroviral in the lab.

Q: What pushed you to pursue your investigation into noni?
A: Basically, it was the basic research done on noni. Then, listening to Dr. Gerson and Dr. Heinicke's tapes really intrigued me. Both of these men are credible scientists. Dr. Heinicke is a fellow Louisvillian whom I could talk to and pick his brain. In talking to him, he showed me a picture of the plant, which rang a bell. As a teenager I used to dig up the root of this plant to make tea for my great uncle, who used it to fix his high blood pressure. And I believe it worked because he lived to be in the nineties before he died of appendicitis, not stroke or heart disease. I have been looking for new nutraceuticals for animals all the time because there are so many animal diseases that are not effective-ly treatable with drugs. In particular, I have been very happy with the fantastic results I've seen using antioxidants to treat animal diseases.

Q: What has been the most fulfilling aspect of your work and expe-rience with noni?
A: My first experience of using noni juice involved saving my cousin's life. She was dying of AIDS and was undergoing treatment with the cocktail of three nasty drugs that wreaked havoc in her organs, all of which had basically failed. She was back to work after only two cases of noni juice. It really blew my mind. Then I started to use it for my own case of debilitating asthma, which I'd had for 25 years. It fixed that in a month. In so doing it also cured my crippling 14-year-old neck and low back pain, for which half a dozen drugs could not give me relief. This is why I lost faith in drug-based therapeutics. Then I used noni to treat my wife's chronic fatigue syndrome and depression that a dozen specialists could not cure. I then helped fix my uncle's BPH (enlarged prostate) and stroke and high blood pressure, my cousin's severe whiplash injury, my niece's jaundice, another cousin's chronic acne, my sister's high cholesterol and high blood pres-

sure, my mother's arthritis, my brother's diabetes mellitus, and a multitude of other health conditions suffered by my friends, neighbors, and co-workers. Then, I finally decided to use it on animals. It worked like a charm; in fact, it has been so effective that I have been using it with every single case I have treated—some 5,000 of them so far. I think I am the first veterinarian to use noni juice on animals in the United States, or for that matter in the world.

Q: What do you think the future holds for noni?
A: I believe that the future of noni is very bright indeed, especially when more people find out what it can do and try it on themselves, their family members, their friends and even their pets. Besides being able to treat already existing conditions, it's great to prevent diseases. I have never seen such a potent nutraceutical.

Q: What do you like best about noni?
A: The things I like best about noni are its potency, its fast action, its safety, and its broad therapeutic spectrum. There is nothing like it on the market place.

Q: What is your favorite story/testimony involving the use of noni?
A: There are so many of them. My favorite, though, is the one involving my cousin. She is still living, despite having terminal AIDS.

Q: Is noni destined to become a household name?
A: Yes. Noni will become a household name because there are already 600,000 people using it only after about three years of worldwide availability. And there is no end in sight. People don't continue to buy and use something unless it works!

Dr. Orlando Pile

"In 1997, I finally decided to become a vegetarian. About the same time I heard on the radio about noni, 'the miracle juice.' Initially, I didn't believe what I heard and decided not to follow up. However, for the next two or three months, I continued to hear over the radio that noni 'does this' and noni 'does that.' So, I finally decided to give it a try.

"On January 1, 1998, I took my first swallow of noni juice. Needless to say, I didn't like the taste. Nevertheless, I was committed to find out how this 'miracle juice' was going to help me—hopefully by lowering my blood pressure and eliminating my anti-hypertensive medications, or by giving me this so-called 'burst' of energy.

"Two months had gone by and I still didn't feel anything. Then, one day while driving with my wife, I was listening to a tape on noni testimonials. 'How can this be?' I thought, 'Everyone is feeling so wonderful after taking noni, including people's pets, and I'm not feeling anything.' At that same moment, my wife asked me about my back condition (referring to my herniated lumbar disk suffered after an auto accident in 1995 and subsequently minimizing my golf playing time). I was so fixed on waiting for this miracle sensation that I never realized my back had stopped hurting. I was so excited that I accepted an invitation to play in a golf tournament in Las Vegas. I took noni before and after playing golf and never had to take one pain killer. For the first time in three years, I was able to play golf without taking a pain pill. I decided to share my experience with my patients in order to hopefully improve their medical conditions.

"I was impressed with the feedback I began to receive. Several patients who had hypertensive blood pressures saw great results. Type II insulin-dependent diabetics were able to lower their insulin doses, and non-insulin-dependent diabetics could either reduce the dose of their medications or even discontinue them altogether. Numerous other patients were able to benefit from taking noni juice. For instance, arthritis patients often reported having less pain in their joints. I also had patients with systemic lupus report positive effects with their pain and other symptoms. Patients with anxiety became more relaxed and slept more soundly. I also had a number of patients report improved bowel and digestive function. A prostate cancer patient experienced a lowering of his PSA level from 16 to 9.12. Finally, I had a terminally ill AIDS patient whose CD4 count increased from 25 to above 200, whose viral load decreased from above 225,000 to 2000, and who saw a healthy weight gain from 78 pounds to 148 pounds in just over one year's time.

"The results on numerous other debilitating disorders continue to astound me. As a practicing internist, I have come to realize that one is able to incorporate the practice of Western medicine with one or more alternative approaches just like noni. Luckily, I have discovered that noni is a powerful and safe therapy for enhancing the health of our patients, our families and most of all, ourselves."

Dr. Joel Murphy

"We have been using Morinda's Tahitian Noni Juice™ for a number of pet health problems. We have had very good success with osteoarthritis, post operative healing, psychoactive disorders, hormonal disorders and for stimulating the immune system. Recently we were presented with a Doberman with grade 2 mast cell cancer that had relapsed twice after surgical removal. Since this cancer is minimally responsive to chemotherapy the owners were searching for alternative approaches.

"We started the patient on noni at a dose of eight ounces divided twice daily. Within 24 hours the tumor shrunk from the size of a baseball to barely palpable. To put things in perspective—this tumor often responds to large doses of cortisone therapy the same way. The remarkable thing is not that the tumor shrunk, but this case demonstrated that the noni juice was as effective as a very large dose of cortisone. This clearly shows that noni has some real therapeutic value. This nice thing about animal studies is that the placebo effect is not a factor."

William Doell, D.O.

Dr. Doell is another doctor who has reported tremendous success among patients using noni to treat their conditions. He writes:

"When I think of all the cases I have treated with noni, there are many that stand out. The first that comes to mind is that of a 43-year-old man who consulted me via telephone, querying whether the analgesic effect of noni would deal with headaches that he was experiencing from his lung cancer that had metastatised to his brain. Though I did not have any experience along those lines, I told him it was worth a try.

"Thus, I told him to take three to four ounces twice daily, always on an empty stomach. After five days of treatment, this man reported to me that the headaches had ceased. He continued on this program for a couple of months, and then returned to his physician for a follow-up visit. The doctor was amazed at his state of health, and asked about the headaches. When told they had ceased, he ordered a CT scan of the patient's brain. The scan revealed no evidence of a tumor! The wise physician decided to check on the primary tumor in the man's lung. It, too, was not visible! This doctor advised the patient to continue doing whatever it was he was doing, and to this day, the patient remains cancer free.

"Of course, there are many, many other examples of noni's powerful health-promoting abilities. Daily, I am amazed at the reports of both my patients and of other health professionals regarding the use of noni juice. In more than 30 years of medicine, I have never witnessed a single product with such universal applicability. In fact, I am convinced that this is the single most valuable health supplement available today!"

Dr. Samuel Kolodney

Dr. Kolodney is one of the growing number of doctors who not only use noni for themselves, but also recommend it to their patients for their ills. He writes:

"My wife, Kelly, and I discovered noni when my sister-in-law Jane brought a small jar of it over to our house. She was very excited and asked us to try it.

"At the time my son was nine months old and was still not sleeping through the night. As a result, we weren't sleeping through the night and hadn't been since he was born. Needless to say we were tired. After taking my first swallow of noni juice I felt my body and mind virtually wake up. I felt the dryness in my eyes go away and Kelly, Jane and I became very excited about the prospect of sharing this powerful and fast-acting product with other people.

"Shortly after, I began to tell some of my regular clients about noni. The ones that decided to try it received good results. I was encouraged by what I saw and began sharing noni with people outside of my chiropractic practice in addition to my regular patients.

"During the past two and a half years many people have reported to me that they recovered from chronic illnesses such as arthritis, high blood pressure, chronic fatigue, joint pain, and diabetes. And the list goes on. However, the first testimonial that truly moved and touched me was from a man with rheumatoid arthritis who proclaimed that noni juice was his 'miracle juice' which had been sent to him by God because it had enabled him to walk when he had previously been confined to sitting because of the constant and severe pain. After two and a half years I still have many miracles reported to me and I witness first-hand many wonderful health changes in people that I have shared noni with.

"My belief in the power of noni to help the body has been fueled both by my personal experiences and those my clients and the extensive review of scientific literature that I have conducted concerning this amazing fruit. I believe that all edible fruits and vegetables can be healing. I also believe that ounce for ounce noni is the most potent healing food on the planet. Continually encouraged by the results I have seen, I want to make this product available not only to those with specific health conditions, but also to everyone, everywhere."

Dru White

Mr. White, one of the first individuals to help in bringing noni to the U.S., describes what noni means to him:

"I believe that when God finished creating the earth—after he was done with his labor—he created one more very special place purely for his own pleasure. He reserved for this last creation some of his most precious and pleasing touches of natural beauty, harmony, and love.

Here, he placed the perfect gift of nature—a simple fruit, called noni, with power to bless the body and lift the spirit. We don't know exactly how or why noni works. He alone knows all its secrets. But we do know that it does work. It has changed the lives of countless people. It contains in it a touch of the divine. Why else would it be so commonly called a 'miracle'?"

Steven Hall, M.D.

Dr. Hall is one of the more well-known physicians who has incorporated noni into his current repertoire of health therapies. He has reported widespread success using noni for a variety of ailments.

"In the fall of 1985, I hurt my back in a trampoline accident, herniating the L5-S1 disc. I received chiropractic treatments but still settled into a chronic pain pattern. Over the next ten years, I tried many treatments, including acupuncture, physical therapy, Hellerwork, glucosamine sulphate, nettle tea, yoga and others. The yoga probably helped more than anything but was unpredictable. Some days, after doing yoga the evening before, I felt better, some days much worse, with shooting pains down my left leg into my left foot. This kept up until the summer of 1995 when my back 'went out' again and I lost the feeling in my left foot. I went for x-rays that showed marked degenerative changes with hypertrophic bone formation at three lumbar levels. I really did not want surgery so continued what I could do, but had to greatly curtail my physical activities.

"In the fall of 1996, a man from whom we had purchased a water filter a few months earlier called Patti, my wife, and told her about noni. She bought two bottles of noni juice from him and requested that I take it. I said 'okay' and started on one ounce twice per day. Almost immediately I found that I was only sleeping about five hours per night. I was expecting to feel run down, but, in actuality, I felt great and was appreciative of the extra two hours per day. Three weeks later, I remember coming home from work and telling Patti that I hadn't thought about my back all that day, which was the first time in over ten years! My spasms were gone. I could still tell that there was arthritis in my back, but gentle stretching started to reliably help instead of sometimes helping, sometimes hurting.

"Three months after starting on the noni juice, feeling returned in my left foot. At first my foot felt like it was just waking up from sitting cross-legged too long—a kind of pins and needles sensation. This lasted about a month, but then complete and normal feeling returned. I noticed other benefits as well, such as a return of my receding gums. When Patti saw the good results with my back, she decided to try noni for herself. Not long after starting to take noni, her chronic problem with migraine headaches was resolved. About this same time, my son, who was a toddler, often fell and hit his head, which several times resulted in a grand mal seizure. We had him evaluated by a pediatric neurologist, whose evaluation was normal. He still wanted to start Aidan on an anti-seizure medicine. All of these medicines can have serious side-effects. I wondered if the noni juice might help Aidan as well. At this point, I started researching noni in earnest.

"I read medical literature, I read ethnobotany literature, I spoke with Dr. Heinicke, the world's foremost expert on noni. I convinced myself that noni juice was completely safe and that, since the specialist couldn't tell us why Aidan was having seizures, anything that we could do to improve the quality of his cellular functioning would be of benefit. We started him on noni juice, one ounce per day. And not only did he like the taste and ask for it often, he hasn't had anymore seizures, nor has he had nearly as many ear infections as did his older siblings. While conducting my investigation into noni, I was very impressed with all of the health problems noni has been used to treat. I have never heard of any other substance that could help alleviate so many problems. Before long, I realized that I had a practice full of people who could benefit from noni. After some soul-searching, I felt comfortable including noni as one of the recommendations I'd make to my patients.

"Right away, I started seeing many interesting results. My practice is composed of people who have generally been to all of the specialists and usually to many alternative practitioners as well and are still not satisfied with their condition. I combine conventional and many natural healing techniques with a model of health and healing that is different from that used by practitioners who focus on treating symptoms. As a result, I've had pretty good results with a wide range of problems not addressed well by conventional medicine, such as autoimmune diseases, allergies, chronic fatigue, fibromyalgia, chronic pain syndromes, etc. But even with all of this, my results are not always 100 percent effective. Sometimes people will improve 80 percent or 60 percent. Quite often, when noni juice was added to their regimen, people would go on to improve 100 percent. I've been using noni juice in my practice now since November of 1996, and I've seen its effects on hundreds and hundreds of people. I have no doubt in my mind that noni juice fills a nutritional niche that we all badly need to have filled. It is unique, versatile and has a beneficial effect on many levels of our well-being."

Del Williams

The following questions and answers are a synthesis from an interview with a reporter and my subsequent personal interview with Del Williams and his wife, Sylvia, in August 1999. Del, who is a retired Delta Airlines pilot, was one of the first people to bring noni to the attention of his family, friends and the world. He told me that he will fly anywhere in the world to tell people about noni juice. In his travels around the globe, he always enjoyed meeting and talking with people about the many health benefits of noni. I would sum up my interview by saying that I am very impressed with Del and Sylvia because they are spiritual people who sincerely care about others.

Q: *Can you share some of your career background before you found out about noni?*
A: I was drafted into military service in 1969. There was a six-year commitment for pilots. I found that many people stayed in the service primarily for financial security in the form of a steady paycheck. I personally felt that people should stay in the military if they had the desire or felt passionate about it.

Q: *What prompted you to be a commercial airline pilot?*
A: I decided to fly as a pilot for Delta airlines because it provided a great income, and a wonderful benefit package, including travel. It left me with the independence to also be a consultant, which I very much enjoy. I needed to do something to help people. I really discovered that I was a people-oriented person.

Q: *How did all this come together with noni?*
A: Taking noni helped me, my family and my friends with a myriad of different health problems. I don't know how it medically works, nor do I really care. I only know that it does, and is safe. I believe noni is God's gift to man I feel passionate about it, and am taking noni juice to help the people of the world. I feel good about it, and the people who take it feel good about it.

Susan List Mike, M.D. and John M. Mike, M.D.

"We are so grateful to have the opportunity to share our thoughts and feelings about this incredible noni juice from French Polynesia. We are both psychiatrists practicing in our holistic medical center and we get exposed to all kinds of nutraceuticals on a daily basis. When we heard about noni juice we were skeptical and yet intrigued by the stories we heard from other physicians, nurses, researchers, and natives of French Polynesia. So we investigated the juice ourselves and shared it with our family and friends first.

"Before starting to take noni for ourselves, we were and still are very healthy; we exercise, eat organic foods, don't drink or smoke and limit our meat intake to mainly fish. I, Susan, noticed that my menstrual cramps were completely gone after two months on the juice. I used to take 800 mg of ibuprofen (that's four tablets) every eight hours for the first two days of my period. After one month on noni, I only used 400 mg and after two months I did not need any ibuprofen. What a relief! My irritability also diminished thanks to the serotonin boost that noni provides by stimulating the pineal gland.

"Our families have also had remarkable results with noni. My mother was relieved of her pain from carpal tunnel syndrome in her wrist after only three weeks on the juice (taking only one ounce a day). She has six grandchildren and three that are under three years old, so she needs full use of her wrists to pick them up and hold them. My uncle experienced relief from chronic gastritis (acid stomach, heartburn). He was in the hospital for a bleeding ulcer two years ago and now he's pain free and eating peppers, spaghetti sauce, or whatever he wants.

"The success with noni only begins with our families. Our patients have found terrific success using noni for their various conditions. We have seen low and high blood pressure normalize, high cholesterol lowered 20 points, diabetes improved to where no pills or less insulin was needed, sleep improved, smoking stopped, anxiety diminished, depression lifted, and energy and motivation increased. We could go on and on. This is a juice from God that helps the body to heal itself and helps people take charge of their own health."

John Wadsworth

Mr. Wadsworth was one of the principal instruments involved in bringing noni out of Tahiti and the South Pacific and into the United States. He currently serves as Vice President of Manufacturing and International Expansion for Morinda, Inc., the first company to bring noni to North America.

"Stephen Story and I were educated at Brigham Young University in food science with a background in nutrition and an emphasis on new product development. Years ago Stephen and I organized a business, the main emphasis of which was to develop new products for network-marketing companies. During this period of time we developed a nutritional bar specifically for the golfer. We thought we would be successful in marketing this bar to hundreds of thousands of golfers in the United States. We invested all the money we had into this project, and after about 120 days in the market place, it was obvious to us that the project was failing, so we closed the business and got back to the basis of developing food.

"It was during this period that I learned of a fruit called *nono*, which was used in Tahiti and surrounding areas to treat various conditions, including diabetes. Consequently, I became more interested in this fruit, and I was eventually able to secure a sample of this product from some natives in Tahiti, which came to our office in St. George. The 'nono' sample was quite interesting. It arrived in a large gallon, wide-mouthed glass jar, which was full of a black liquid. As I looked closer, I noticed there was more than just juice: there were also small fruits, some leaves and a branch. I also noticed that the lid on the jar was rusty, and there was a piece of newspaper between the lid and the jar to act as a seal.

"Needless to say, this was a very crude sample. I didn't quite know what to do with it at first, so I pushed it over to the side of my desk. A few days later I came into the office and noticed the crude sample of fruit sitting in the corner of my desk, so I decided to open it. As I slid up toward the jar and began to remove the lid, I heard some pressure release from the bottle. From the sound of this pressure I immediately knew that there was some gas being formed, probably from fermentation. As this gas was released, the room was immediately filled with an indescribable stench. It was so bad that I left the office, closing the door behind me. When I returned to the office, I noticed the stench still lingering, so I fanned the door for several minutes to clear the air. I didn't know what to do with this crude and stinky sample, but because of the circumstances that Steve and I were under, I felt the need to pursue the investigation into this 'nono.'

"Consequently, I approached several individuals who were known diabetics, and asked if they would be willing to take the juice on a trial basis to see if it would help normalize their blood sugar. In each case, as they smelled a sample of the juice, their response was a definite 'no.' Finally, I approached a young man 18 years of age who had Type I diabetes. After smelling the juice, he told me, 'I will take this juice only if you will take it with me.' Up to this point I had not tasted the juice, nor did I have any interest in doing so, mainly because I didn't have diabetes and didn't think I would receive any benefit from taking it.

"So I set up a schedule for us to take the nono juice—at 6 a.m. each morning and at 7 p.m. each night, as instructed by a Tahiti native. I still remember the morning that was scheduled for the first administration of the product. It was a Monday, and the previous day I had come down with a cold which hit me very hard. Because the aroma was so strong, I was reluctant to take this ugly, stinky juice for the first time. Because of my reluctance, our young subject was also reluctant. So we put some juice on two large tablespoons and swallowed it simultaneously, as though we were looking in the mirror at each other. As soon as the juice entered my mouth, my first thought was that the smell was not that bad. The flavor of the juice was so repugnant that I ran to the sink and grabbed a glass of water, using it as a chaser.

"Well, we eventually got over the smell and taste, and together we took this juice religiously every morning and every night for approximately four weeks. While taking the product we tested the blood sugar level of our subject regularly, and recorded the results. At the end of the study and in analyzing the results, our conclusion was that it did not affect this young man in any way. However, I noticed that when I took the juice it helped relieve the symptoms of the cold that I had contracted just days before. But because the results of the test showed no promise to relieve the symptoms of this young man's diabetes, I once again sealed the jar, put it on a top shelf, and tried to find another project to pursue. Several weeks after the conclusion of this trial, a woman came to the office and reported that she had a cold and couldn't get rid of the symptoms. She reported that she had been to the doctor and had taken medication, but could not relieve the symptoms. This young woman asked if we had anything that could help her with this cold. As she said this, I remembered how this juice had affected me as I took it. I responded by telling her we might have something, and asked her to leave the office while I prepared a sample because I did not want her to smell it. I prepared a sample in a very clean jar, enough for a ten-day supply. I then presented this sample to her, giving specific instructions on how and when she should take the juice. I told her to come back in eight days so we could discuss the results.

"She returned as instructed, and reported that she had taken the product as directed. I asked her if she felt it had relieved the symptoms of her cold. Her response was that although she did not have the symptoms anymore, she did not know whether or not the 'nono' had helped. However, she was very excited to report that she felt it helped the arthritis in her knees. She explained that she was a walker and had not been able to walk for many weeks because of the pain in her knees. While she was on this juice it helped to relieve the pain in her knees so she could walk. This sparked some interest, so I began to study the demographics of the population who has arthritis, and determined that if this juice actually did offer some relief to those people, we could build a business.

"My next trial was with six elderly individuals. These individuals had arthritis, and each was willing to participate in a short study. A sample of product was given to each individual with instructions on how and when to take it. They were told to record their observations while taking the juice. After the designated four-week term, something almost completely unexpected happened. Each one of these individuals, in reporting their findings, asked for more juice. This was all I needed to hear. I had smelled the juice and had taken it myself, and knew that if they wanted more, it wasn't because they were taking it as a refreshment beverage. It was because it had helped them with their specific health problems.

"These were very positive results, so I thought that maybe we should try this same study with a Type II diabetic. We soon found a qualified patient, who had a blood sugar level of 210. Again, I prepared a sample and presented the sample to him with instructions. In eight days this individual returned, reporting that without any change in life style or diet, his blood sugar was reduced to 110. This news gave us enough excitement and information that we decided to continue to pursue this project, so I made preparations to travel to Tahiti to do further research.

"When arriving in Tahiti the first order of business was to find out more about the history of this product. I began by interviewing people on the street. After finding an interpreter, I began asking the question to people we met, 'What can you tell me about the nono fruit plant?' The response to this question was quite interesting to me. Whenever I asked this question to a native, they had a story to tell me. The story was of themselves, their grandfather, aunt, or sister. The illnesses mentioned in these stories in which 'nono' assisted in their recovery, ranged from cold sores to menstrual cramps, back pain, headaches, cuts and abrasions, diabetes, arthritis, cancer, etc. I was astonished at the stories I was being told. I wasn't sure whether I should believe the far-reaching claims. Up to this point I felt that it helped with arthritis and diabetes, but that was the extent of my experience. On the other hand, I noticed that whenever I asked a person whose lineage was from France, they knew nothing about the fruit or the plant. I soon realized that the French use western medicine and they were not familiar with the traditional healing practices of the natives.

"This led me to research out some of the native medicine people practicing the natural remedies passed down from generation to generation. In interviewing these people, I learned that the natives had used this product for literally hundreds and hundreds of years. I was also able to review their medicine books, which contained recipes of natural remedies written hundreds of years before and handed down from generation to generation. In reviewing these books carefully, I noticed the word 'nono' in almost every recipe. Through further investigation, it was made known to me that this product was not only used for over a thousand years, but was also used to relieve the symptoms of most every ailment known to the natives. This information led me to further examine how the natives prepared this fruit for administration to the sick.

"So, I looked to the libraries for further information and found some writings with regard to the history of nono, but none that were very extensive. I met with members of the government specializing in botany and plant life of the islands, and found additional evidence that what I learned from the medicine people was true. I also found that the government of the United States approved nono as a food in the early 1940s. During World War II, the military established a base on the island of Bora Bora. In setting up this base they researched the native fruits and plants, and realized the natives ate this nono in times of famine, and thus approved this and other fruits and vegetables native to the area as a food.

"During this first trip to Tahiti, my discoveries and findings were extremely interesting and supported the notion that nono could provide significant health benefits. I soon returned to Tahiti to further my investigation and to see if there was enough fruit to support a large company. In this research, I learned that the 'nono' plant is quite remarkable. It grows throughout the Pacific both in acid and basic soils. It does not have a season, and produces fruit year round. On a given tree you will see fruit in all stages of maturity.

"In visiting Tahiti and other nearby islands, I discovered that although there was fruit on each island, I didn't believe there was enough fruit to support a large company. I also learned that when the fruit falls on the ground it gives off a bad aroma, so in many cases the natives would control the growth of the tree by cutting it down because it smelled so bad. I discussed with the people my desire to gather the fruit and take it to market, the typical response was either disbelief or laughter. Even though the natives used the juice from the fruit to relieve symptoms of many ailments, they felt that the odor and the flavor were so bad that no one would actually pay money for the juice. I was becoming quite concerned that there was not enough fruit. I kept hearing that I would need to go to the Marquesas Islands to find fruit in plenty.

"In making preparations to go to Marquesas (part of French Polynesia), which is a group of five or six islands 1,000 miles north of Tahiti, I found that travel to these islands was very expensive. In fact an airfare was three times more expensive from Tahiti to Marquesas, as opposed to Los Angeles from Tahiti. Because the failed golf business Steve and I started, I was short on cash, so I was quite concerned about spending the money to go to Marquesas. I further learned that I would need to take two interpreters with me, one that knew the local dialect as well as Tahitian, and one that knew Tahitian as well as English. Because the expense of this trip was becoming so large, I asked my interpreter to call ahead and ask some people that he knew if there was a lot of 'nono' to make the trip successful. He reported that the people in Marquesas were saying that there was plenty of 'nono' and that they were very excited for us to come over, gather it all up, put it in a box, and take it back with us.

"I thought this was an odd response, so I asked him to go back and confirm it. Each time his report was the same. After three reports being the same, I figured we better go.

"I remember the day of our travel was a beautiful day. We arrived at the airport early in the morning to board our plane bound for Nuka Hiva. As the boarding call was made for our plane, I was very excited to take this new adventure. The plane, which was an old plane, was very small with a propeller on each wing. We departed the island of Tahiti, and headed northward to the Marquesas. The plane was very loud and vibrated noisily. We flew low, I suppose because either the plane couldn't get high, or because it wasn't pressurized.

"The flight, because of the noise and vibration, was exhausting. Despite the inconveniences, we arrived on the dry side of the island, opposite of the town which we were headed to. The only thing on this dry side of the island was a little hut right at the airport. In walking into this small hut, I asked Tom where our ride was. Up to this time, when I asked Tom to make preparations for lodging and transportation, I was thinking the Hilton Hotel and a stretch limousine. Tom went over to the other side of the hut and was conversing with some people. After several minutes of waiting he came over to me and said, 'John we have our ride. It's out front.' We walked out front and to my surprise the only thing out there was an old open air, rusted-out jeep, which looked to me like it barely survived World War II. As we arrived at the jeep, I noticed that the back seat didn't have any padding so I wanted to sit in the front seat. Tom also wanted to sit in the front seat, so he convinced me to sit in the back by saying that because he knew the language and could speak with the driver, it was best if he sat in front. The other interpreter whom I brought found a ride with a friend, so I sat in the back as our jeep headed for our destination.

"Now it rains a lot in Nuka Hiva, and this beautiful island is a mountain that shoots out of the ocean and towers over 10,000 feet above sea level. There are no roads around the island so you have to go over the top of the mountain to get to the other side. The roads are not paved, so due to the high amount of rainfall, they are filled with ruts and switchbacks. Needless to say, it was a very rough ride. I went from a shaking plane to a very bumpy jeep without a padded seat, and again it took over four hours to drive from the airport to town.

"Upon arriving at our destination, I was very tired. We were to stay with a family whose home was a very small, one-room hut. I noticed that they hung a sheet in the middle, which created a division with us sleeping on one side of the sheet and the family sleeping on the other. It was very hot, there were bugs flying around and I was very tired and frustrated.

"Soon after our arrival, Tom engaged in conversation with the owners of the home. As they conversed, I heard the word *nono*, which I was very familiar with. I also heard the word *noni*, which seemed familiar but I wasn't sure of the meaning. After several minutes of conversation, Tom came to me and said, 'John we have a problem.' I wondered what problem we could have that was greater than the airplane and jeep ride. So I said, 'What's the problem? I'm ready.' He said, 'Well, each time I called ahead and asked if there was enough nono they reported there was a lot of nono. John, there is a lot of nono here, but I just discovered that the word *nono* in Marquesas is a little bug similar to a mosquito. It bites, and if you get enough bites it will make you sick. These people were very excited for us to come and collect all the "nono" and take it back with us because it is such a nuisance. The word that describes the fruit is *noni*. So there has been a bit of miscommunication. The word *nono* in Tahiti is the fruit, and the word *noni* in Tahiti is the bug, and in Marquesas it's the opposite and I didn't realize that.'

"Well, needless to say, this news was devastating to me. After hearing this news I was filled with an enormous depression and responded to Tom by saying, 'I'm really not interested in finding bugs. I've spent all this money to come over here. Now I just want to forget all of the research on this nono and go home. I will start working on a project that is more familiar to me. I will create a product that is more known and accepted among Americans. Let's just go home.' His response was even more depressing. 'That's another problem,' he said. 'The plane for us to return to Tahiti will not come back for three more days.'

"After hearing this response, I didn't know what to do. The next morning, after having been able to think it over, I decided to take advantage of those three days and see if there was any way to salvage the trip and possibly the project.

"The first thing I did was make preparations to have a town meeting to visit with all of the farmers in the area, hoping that I could convince them to start growing this noni plant to ensure our supply. After an hour and a half of trying to convince them to grow this fruit, their response was basically laughter.

"For two and a half days we drove around the island in search of noni. In our search, I really was not impressed and felt that there was about as much noni in the islands of Marquesas as there was in the other islands I had visited earlier. At this point I was becoming very depressed because there was not enough fruit in my estimation to supply a large company. The last evening that we were there, as we were returning back to town after a long day of searching for noni, we stopped on the top of a ridge to rest our legs. As I stepped out of the jeep I was taken back by the beautiful sunset that was on the horizon. The sun was just setting over the mountains in the west. It was that time of day when you can look directly at the sun and see it pulsating. The sky was filled with this beautiful orange, red, calming reflection. The sight was so beautiful, I was drawn toward it and walked to the other side of the road to the edge of the ravine. I was moved by the beauty of the scene, and noticed that my eyes were drawn by the rays of the sun to the valley below. As I looked to the valley beneath my feet, I noticed that the rays of the sun were accenting the leaves of some trees below. I immediately realized that these plants were noni plants, and upon identifying them, I further noticed that the valley was filled with the plant. As I was struck with this beauty, a very powerful impression came to me. This impression was real then, and it's real to me today. The impression was simply this: This product has been preserved from the world, and now is the time to take it to the world. It will bless the lives of millions and millions of people and it will also bless the lives of the people in Tahiti.

"This impression came to me with power and conviction, and in my mind, I could see many different people taking this juice, all of which had different colors of skin and different shape of eyes. They were from nations all over the world. Each time I think of this impression, my body tingles with some of the same sensations that I had as I stood on the side of that mountain looking at the setting sun. This powerful influence came to me at the most depressing time in my life and definitely at the most depressing time in my career. I wanted to quit, I wanted to do something easier. I was tired of people laughing at me telling me it couldn't be done. Up to this point it was a job, but after this impression it became a part of me and I couldn't stop despite the laughter and disparaging comments. I couldn't stop, nor will I stop until this vision is completed.

"At the time I really didn't realize the significance of the impression that the noni fruit had been preserved. It was not a secret. The natives knew about this plant for thousands of years and were willing to share it with anyone that asked. Yet the world did not know about it. Well, this experience gave me strength to continue. On my way home from my trip, I stopped at the University of Hawaii to do further research. I found the work of Dr. Ralph Heinicke and Anne Hirazumi, and others who had done research on this plant and its medicinal values. This research was very exciting to come across. You see, at this point we knew we had a good product, we knew it helped people, but we didn't know how or why it worked. This research, particularly Dr. Ralph Heinicke's documents, described to us a mechanism to answer these questions. I returned to Tahiti several additional times to discover a process which would allow us to provide this juice at a commercial level, and yet still have the same medicinal value as when the natives prepared it. The process which was discovered, and which we use today, is a process which provides this juice the same way that the natives have used it for thousands and thousands of years.

"During my discovery, I traveled to other islands throughout the Pacific to see if there was enough fruit. In my travels, I discovered that the best fruit is in French Polynesia. In French Polynesia, these islands are untouched. They are virgin territories if you will, with very little population. The water is pure and the air is clean. I found that the fruit there is larger, the trees are larger, the leaves are larger, and the trees bear more fruit.

"After finally identifying the process that would ensure a quality product, we began to present this product to successful network marketing companies. It was not our intent to start a new company, but our intent was to place this product with a successful network marketing company and enter into a contract where we could provide the raw ingredients.

"As I stated earlier, we had developed products for many network-marketing companies, so it was very easy for us to get in and see some of the most successful companies in the industry. Since we were well acquainted with these companies, we identified five companies that we thought would offer the most potential with this product. We were shocked at the response of each company that we took the product to. Each company rejected the product due to the notion of marketing a stinky food from the middle of the Pacific. The reason for my shock was because I knew how powerful the product was. We provided ample information for them to make an educated decision, yet they had no interest.

"So, we built a business plan and started approaching people with regard to funding a new company. Steve and I were close associates with Kelly Olsen. At this time Kelly was employed by another network marketing company as the Vice President of Marketing. Because of our close association with him, we knew of his experience and tremendous aptitude with regard to creating and promoting marketing plans. We met with him several times to encourage him to join us. In one of these meetings we shared the all-natural unflavored noni juice with Kelly. After his observance of the odor and the flavor, his response was that we should flavor the product, and if we did we would be more successful. In our efforts to convince him otherwise, I reminded him of a company he worked for which had a product of similar odor and flavor, and that sold more than a quarter of a billion dollars a year. His response was, 'What do you think they would have sold if it tasted good?' That statement convinced Steve and I to flavor the product.

"All this was happening at the same point that we were introduced to Kerry and Kim Asay. We initiated a meeting with them, which was quite interesting. We then told them of the story of the Polynesian people and how noni had helped them for thousands of years. We discussed the ailments and illnesses against which history showed this product to be effective. We gave them much of the research that we found, including Anne Hirazumi and Dr. Ralph Heinicke's findings. The meeting was a very short but powerful engagement. Kerry reports that during the meeting when he was listening to the story of the Polynesian people and heard the word noni, that it touched his heart. He said it was like someone opened his chest, grabbed his heart, and massaged it. Apparently, Kerry and Kim had been looking for a project to get involved with for many years. In their search they prayed for guidance and they looked at many different projects. This one felt different than any others they had discovered. Kerry reports that when they left our first meeting together, that he and Kim discussed this feeling and both felt that this project was right for them. We soon negotiated an agreement between us and formed Morinda, Inc. in 1995.

"Since then, we have organized operations in sixteen markets throughout the world, and we expect the growth to continue.

"One of the reasons for our success is that the product works, and the people need it. We believe that this project is greater than we are. We believe that it is a gift from the great creator who has placed it here upon this earth to benefit mankind. I don't know why I was on that mountain on that day, but because I was there and had that experience, I now feel a responsibility and a charge to continue our efforts."

Safe and Effective
Use of Noni

I AM OFTEN asked about the best ways to use noni. Which is the most effective form, juice or capsule? How much is enough? What times during the day are best to drink noni juice, and how many times a day? Is it safe to use with prescription drugs? Are there any side effects from using noni? Can I take too much noni? These, among others, certainly are all legitimate questions that reflect real concerns. The truth is, we don't have definitive answers to all these questions, though there is mounting evidence that provides important clues that can help us use noni more safely and effectively.

In my research of noni, I have often faced the question as to what form of noni is best. While noni juice was the first form of noni to arrive in North America, several other forms, most notably freeze-dried capsules, have also been developed. So, to answer the question as to which is best, I can only answer that the overwhelming majority of the data that I collected from doctors and noni users, as well as the scientific research surrounding the noni fruit, have involved the use of the juice from the noni fruit harvested from the islands of French Polynesia (Tahiti and surrounding islands). In addition, because the harvesting, processing and packaging processes all vary from company to company, it is difficult to establish a standard for serving amounts and frequency of consumption. Consequently, in the following discussion of safety and usage issues concerning noni, keep in mind that I am generally referring to Tahitian Noni Juice™.

"How Much Noni Should I Use?"

Table 1 lists the recommended test, loading, therapeutic, and maintenance/preventive serving amounts of noni juice in ounces, to be used for both adults and children. Animals under 100 pounds should be given the children's serving, while animals weighing more than 100 pounds should be given the adult serving. A test serving, which is often helpful in determining if the individual is sensitive to noni, can be tried before proceeding to the loading amount. This test amount should consist of two teaspoons of noni juice per day for three days. Nearly everyone who uses noni (more than 99 percent) tolerates it. However, there is an extremely small percentage of users (less than 1 percent) who experience allergic reactions. If you develop a rash, hives, wheezing, or swelling in the neck/face, stop taking noni immediately, as you may be in this small group of those who are allergic to noni.

Originally, according to Dr. Heinicke, there need be no serving size adjustment for humans as to weight because proxeronine from noni juice is stored in and released by the liver. However, in our survey of more than 10,000 noni juice users, better results were obtained for both men and women when an additional one-half ounce was added for every additional 50 pounds over 250 pounds.

And what are the best times of the day to drink noni juice? Ideally, noni juice should be consumed just before breakfast and just before dinner. (However, if this schedule cannot be followed, it is better to use noni whenever possible rather than not taking it at all.) It is also important to remember that noni exerts its positive effects quickly in many people, and most people experience results within days to weeks. But you should commit to using noni for six months before deciding how much it helps.

If you feel that during months two through seven you are not getting optimal improvement, increase your daily intake by an additional one-half ounce of noni juice for seven days, dividing the total serving size between morning, noon, and evening. Increase the total serving every seven days by the same amount until you obtain the desired results or until you drink a bottle or more of noni per day (very few people need more than this).

Test Serving: 3 Days

	TEASPOONS OF NONI JUICE
Adult (over 16 years)	
Before breakfast	1
Before dinner	1
Child (under 16 years)	
Before breakfast	1

Loading Serving: Month 1

	OUNCES OF NONI JUICE
Adult (over 16 years)	
Before breakfast	2
Before dinner	2
Child (under 16 years)	
Before breakfast	1
Before dinner	1

Therapeutic Serving: Month 2 through Month 6

	OUNCES OF NONI JUICE
Adult (over 16 years)	
Before breakfast	2
Before dinner	1
Child (under 16 years)	
Before breakfast	1
Before dinner	1/2

Maintenance/Prevention Serving: Month 7 and After

	OUNCES OF NONI JUICE
Adult (over 16 years)	
Before breakfast	1
Before dinner	1
Child (under 16 yrs.)	
Before breakfast	1

Table 12.1: **Test, loading, therapeutic and maintenance serving amounts of noni juice for humans and animals. Note that animals over 100 lbs. use the adult serving; animals under 100 lbs. use the child serving.**

Some people may wonder about noni's interactions with other drugs, food supplements or medical procedures. While due caution should be given, there is no evidence that noni is toxic in any manner, nor is it dangerous to use with other drugs or natural supplements. In fact, I, as well as many other health professionals, have received numerous reports indicating that noni can actually enhance the action of other health-promoting agents.

In addition, there is evidence supporting the notion that noni may also be used by pregnant and/or lactating women. However, as I have previously stated, before starting to take noni or any food supplement it is wise to consult with your physician and/or health-care provider.

Commonly Asked Questions Concerning Noni

Over the last few years, I have been asked numerous questions regarding noni and its reported therapeutic capabilities. Taking into consideration the fact that our knowledge of noni is continually expanding, the following are some of the most common questions put to me concerning noni, as well as the answers I generally give.

Q: *Does noni really work?*
A: Simply stated, yes. Again, I believe that noni can be taken by anyone, anywhere, and can benefit most people for most conditions most of the time.

Q: *Is noni safe?*
A: Yes—it has been used safely by hundreds of thousands of people worldwide for thousands of years. This includes pregnant and lactating women, children, the elderly and those in-between.

Q: *What are the side effects from taking noni?*
A: For most people, there are no side effects from using noni, even when taken in large doses. For the few (less than 1 percent) who are allergic to noni fruit, they can experience a rash, itching, and/or diar-

rhea. Within 24 hours after discontinuing noni, the allergic side effects usually disappear. Non-allergic side effects appear in less than 2 percent and may consist of slight belching, mild diarrhea, gas, and/or nausea. These side effects are significantly decreased or alleviated within 24 hours after the noni serving size is decreased (usually to about half the current amount).

Q: Who should use noni?
A: Again, I believe that noni can be used by anyone, anywhere, and can help most people with most health conditions.

Q: Specifically, with what conditions can noni supplementation help?
A: There are numerous ailments for which noni has been used over the years. Historical use and current data show it has been used effectively for numerous major health conditions, including cancer, hypertension, diabetes, arthritis, chronic pain, various types of infections, rheumatic ailments, sinusitis, ulcers, depression, skin disorders, lupus, fibromyalgia, herpes, hepatitis, digestive/eliminatory problems, heart disease, HIV, and anxiety. Of course, there are a host of other ailments—too many to list here—for which noni has been used effectively.

Q: How is noni able to help treat so many different ailments?
A: This question deserves more of an explanation than I can give here. However, when explained in basic terms, noni has been shown to possess several specific health-promoting characteristics, all of which contribute to its effectiveness against a variety of conditions. One of these characteristics is that of being an adaptogen. Just like it sounds, an adaptogen helps the body "adapt" to the problems present through a number of processes. Research indicates that noni may help fight disease at a cellular level, aiding malfunctioning or "sick" cells by helping them regain their normal function. This in turn allows the body to eventually reverse one or more conditions. For more in-depth explanations as to how noni may help treat such an impressive array of health conditions, refer to chapters 4–9.

Q: *How much noni is adequate?*
A: Because we are all individuals with different physical needs, the amount of noni required to help achieve the desired result varies. A basic rule of thumb is to take as much as is needed to achieve the desired effect. In general though, most people have experienced at least some benefit by following the serving guidelines found in Table 1 of this chapter.

Q: *How long should I use noni?*
A: Again, because we all have varying needs, you can take noni for as long as necessary to make you feel better. In my survey of more than 10,000 noni users, of the 78 percent of all people who reported that noni helped them in some way, 95 percent said that they experienced benefits within 3 months. However, many people report success within just a few days to a few weeks. Additionally, you ought to use noni for as long as it makes you feel better.

Q: *How pure is noni?*
A: This question is difficult to answer, mainly because of the fact that there are several companies that now manufacture a noni product. In addition, there is not much research regarding the purity of different commercial products, so it is easy to assume that the purity and quality of each product may vary from company to company. However my research findings, which suggest that noni juice is, in general terms, extremely safe, were done principally on data gathered from noni fruit harvested from more than 100 different French Polynesian islands. Two qualified independent laboratories also tested and found noni juice from these islands to be free from over 600 possible contaminants.

My Conclusion: Start Using Noni Now!

As I discussed in earlier sections of this book, our country, and Western health care in general, is currently undergoing a virtual revolution in terms of how we take care of our health and well-being. There is a definite movement towards a more holistic approach to solving health problems and regaining vibrant and optimal health.

As part of this movement has come the recognition that nutrition plays a primary role in maintaining good health. However, for various reasons concerning dietary habits and other lifestyle factors, it may be difficult for many of us to consume the nutrients necessary to achieve optimal health. That is why supplementing with natural products—like noni—can often play a key role in successfully treating already-present health conditions and preventing others.

In writing this book, I have attempted to provide a definitive picture of the tropical healer noni and the exciting and promising information regarding its use as a safe and effective health-promoting agent. Used for centuries among various cultures around the world to fight a multitude of health conditions, noni is now gaining a strong foothold in our own culture as a safe and powerful health supplement.

Just like myself, there are literally tens of thousands of Americans and others worldwide who, though initially may have been skeptics, are now firm believers in the remarkable ability of noni to alleviate a number of ailments and disorders, prevent the onset of others and help you achieve a new level of health.

ENDNOTES

Chapter 1

1. Abbott, I.A., and C. Shimazu. "The Geographic Origin of the Plants most Commonly Used for Medicine by Hawaiians." *Journal of Ethnopharmacology* 14 (1985): 213-22.
2. Drury, Colonel Heber. *Useful Plants of India, with Notice of Their Chief Value in Commerce, Medicine and the Arts,* 2nd edition. William H. Allen And Co. London, 1873: 296.
3. "The Wealth of India." *Council of Scientific and Industrial Research* 6 (1962): 423.
4. Rock, Joseph. "The Indigenous Trees of the Hawaiian Islands." Published under patronage; Honolulu, 1913: 467.
5. Kepler, A.K. *Hawaiian Heritage Plants.* Honolulu: Oriental Publishing, 1983.
6. Morton, Julia. "The Ocean-Going Noni, or Indian Mulberry (*Morinda citrifolia*) and some of Its 'Colorful' Relatives. *Economic Botany* 3 (1992): 241-256.
7. Benthall, 1946.
8. Dalziel, 1937: in *Medicinal Plants in Tropical West Africa,* by Oliver Bever.
9. Burkill, I.H. *A Dictionary of the Economic Products of the Malay Peninsula.* 2 (1966): 1518.

Chapter 3

1. Hirazumi, Anne. "Antitumor Studies of a Traditional Hawaiian Medicinal Plant, Morinda citrifolia (Noni), In Vitro and In Vivo." Doctoral dissertation, summary: 1997.

Chapter 4

1. Blakeslee, S. "Surprise Discovery: Hemoglobin Has Bigger Role." *The New York Times,* March 21, 1996: A1-22.
2. Kolata, G. "Key signal of cells found to be a common gas." *The New York Times,* July 2,

1991: C1 & C6.

3. Park, K.G.M., Hayes, P.D., Garlick, P.J., Swell, H., and Eremin, O. "Stimulation of lymphocyte natural cytotoxicity by L-arginine." *The Lancet* 337 (1991): 645-646.

4. Hirazumi, Anne. "Antitumor Studies of a Traditional Hawaiian Medicinal Plant, Morinda citrifolia (Noni), In Vitro and In Vivo." Doctoral dissertation, University of Hawaii: 1997.

5. Levand, Oscar. "Some Chemical Constituents of Morinda citrifolia L. (Noni)." Doctoral thesis, part I, University of Hawaii; 1963: 2.

6. Kumar, et al. In *Basic Pathology*, 6th ed. W.B. Saunders Company, Philadelphia: 1997.

Chapter 5

1. Hirazumi, Anne. "Antitumor Studies of a Traditional Hawaiian Medicinal Plant, Morinda citrifolia (Noni), In Vitro and In Vivo." Doctoral dissertation, University of Hawaii: 1997.

2. Wang, Mian-Ying, M.D. "Chemopreventive Activity of Tahitian Noni Juice in C57BL-6 Mice." (unpublished at time of printing), abstract, UIC College of Medicine at Rockford, Dept. of Biomedical Sciences, 1999.

3. Rennick et al. "Interleukin-10: an overview." *Progress in Growth Factor Research* 4 (1992): 207-227.

4. Hirazumi, 1997.

5. Block, G. "Epidemiologic evidence regarding vitamin C and cancer." *American Journal of Clinical Nutrition* 54 (1991): 1310S-14S.

Chapter 6

1. Solomon, N. and C.C. Carpenter, I.L. Bennett and A.M. Harvey. "Schmidt's syndrome (thyroid and adrenal insufficiency) and co-existence of diabetes mellitus." *Diabetes* 14 (1965): 300.

Chapter 7

1. McDougall, John A. *The McDougall Program for a Healthy Heart*. New York: Dutton, 1996: 215-16.

2. Hirazumi, A., Rursawa, E., Chou, S.C., and Hokama, Y. "Anticancer activity of Morinda citrifolia (Noni) on intraperitoneally implanted Lewis Lung carcinoma in syngeneic mice." *Proc. West Pharmacology Society* 37 (1994): 145-46.

3. Nakaki, T., Hishikawa, K., Suzuki, H., Saruta, T., and Kato, R. (1990): "L-Arginine-induced hypotension." *The Lancet*, 336, 696.

4. Hishikawa, K., Nakaki, T., Suzuki, H., Kato, R., and Saruta, T. "L-arginine as an Antihypertensive agent." *Journal of Cardiovascular Pharmacology Supplement* 20 (1992): S196-197.

5. Osilesi, O., et al. "Blood pressure and plasma lipids during ascorbid acid supplementation in borderline hypertensive and normotensive adults." *Nutrition Research* 11 (1991): 405-12.

6. Little, Pl, et al. "A controlled trial of a low-sodium, low-fat, high-fiber diet in treated hyperensive patients: the efficacy of multiple dietary intervention." *Postgraduate Medical Journal* 66 (1990): 616-21.

7. Moore, T. "The role of dietary electrolytes in hypertension." *Journal of American College Nutrition* 8 (1989): 68S-80S.

8. Salonen, J. et al. "Blood pressure, dietary fats, and antioxidants." *American Journal of American Nutrition* 48 (1988): 1226-32.

9. Yamagami, T. "Bioenergetics in clinical medicine: Studies on coenzyme Q10 and essential hypertension." *Res. Commun. Chem. Pathol. Pharmacol.* 11 (1975): 273.

Chapter 8

1. Khalsa, Dharma Singh. *The Pain Cure.* New York: Warner Books, 1999: 4-10.

2. Tran, Gary. Personal communication, 1997.

3. Cox, Paul. Personal communication, 1997)

4. Dicks, Richard. Personal communication, 1997.

5. Khalsa, 228.

6. Ibid., 229.

7. Walsh, N.D. et al. "Analgesic Effectiveness of D-phenylalanine in chronic pain patients." *Arch Phys Med Rehabil* 7 (1986): 436-39.

Chapter 9

1. Chronic Fatigue and Immune Dysfunction Association of America. *The CFIDS Chronicle* July/August, 1999.

2. "Psychological Symptoms in Chronic Fatigue and Juvenile Rheumatoid Arthritis," *Pediatrics* May 1999.

3. "Stigma and Chronic Fatigue Syndrome." *Chronic Fatigue Syndrome* 5 (1999).

4. Teitelbaum, Jacob, M.D. *From Fatigued to Fantastic!* Garden City Park, N.Y.: Avery Publishing Group/ 1996: 6.

5. Hyde, B.M., ed. *The Clinical and Scientific Basis of Myalgic Encephalitis and Chronic Fatigue Syndrome.* Ottawa: Nightingale Research Foundation, 1992.

6. Theodosakis, Jason, et al. *The Arthritis Cure.* New York: St. Martin's Press, 1997: 149.

7. Morton, Julia. "The Ocean-Going Noni, or Indian Mulberry (Morinda citrifolia, Rubiaceae) and Some of Its 'Colorful' Relatives, *Economic Botany* 46 (1992): 241-56.

8. Bushnell, O.A., et al. "The Antibacterial Properties of Some Plants Found in Hawaii." *Pacific Science* 4 (1950): 167-83.

9. Levand, O. "Some Chemical Constituents of Morinda citrifolia." In unpublished doctor-

al dissertation from the University of Hawaii, 1963.

10. Hirazumi, Anne. "Antitumor Studies of a Traditional Hawaiian Medicinal Plant, Morinda citrifolia (Noni), In Vitro and In Vivo." Doctoral dissertation, University of Hawaii: 1997.

11. Duncan, S.H., Flint, H.J., and Stewart, C.S. "Inhibitory activity of gut bacteria against *Escherichia coli* 0157 mediated by dietary plant metabolites." *FEMS Microbiology Letter,* 164 (1998): 283-88.

12. Gary Tran, personal communication.

INDEX

Abbott, Isabelle 47, 70
abdominal gas 192
adaptogen 55, 283
adrenaline 157, 164
AIDS 167, 216, 256
ALA 177
alcohol 29, 64, 68, 98–99, 190, 207
alcoholics 208
alfalfa 177
allergic reactions 280
allergies 192, 263
amino acids 72, 101, 110, 125, 142, 169, 200
angina 62, 139, 169
animals 21–22, 82, 84–85, 99, 167–168, 217, 219, 222, 244–245, 250, 254–256, 280–281
ankylosing spondylitis 172, 205, 212
anxiety 37, 126, 151, 163, 165, 170–171, 189–190, 193, 201, 216, 226, 257, 265, 283
arginine 65, 67, 144
arthritis 20, 23–24, 30–31, 33, 35, 37–38, 43, 47–48, 50–52, 57, 88, 96, 150, 160, 166–169, 173–174, 177–179, 184, 187, 202–206, 208–212, 217–219, 221–222, 228–229, 231, 233–236, 244, 252, 256–257, 260–261, 268–269, 283, 289
Asay, Kerry 9, 42, 52, 248
Asay, Kim 9, 42, 245, 249, 275
Bacillus subtilis 213

back pain 160, 166–167, 169, 205, 209, 255, 268
beta cells 110–112, 114–116, 119, 121–122, 124
bladder infections 192, 215
blood sugar 107, 109–111, 113, 117–122, 124, 126, 128, 266–268
boils 169, 213–214
bone spurs 228
brain 21, 24, 49, 60, 62–63, 139, 162–164, 170–171, 177–178, 191–192, 194, 196, 198, 201, 221, 235–238, 248, 255, 259
bromelain 56–57, 59–60, 71, 242–244, 248
bursitis 169, 206–207, 212
caffeine 149, 171
cancer 3, 12, 30–31, 38, 45–48, 50–52, 55, 57, 65–67, 71, 77, 79–87, 89–91, 93–97, 99–103, 107, 138, 160, 166, 169, 183, 186–187, 200, 208, 218, 220, 235, 237–238, 244, 250, 253, 257–259, 269, 283, 288
    use of noni with 45–46, 80–81
    history of 82
    xeronine and 87
    nitric oxide and 87
    immune system and 82-89
carbohydrates 49, 108–110, 124
carbon monoxide 171
carcinogenesis 81
cardiovascular system 33, 64–65, 135,

138, 141, 143–145, 148, 152, 220
carpal tunnel syndrome 169, 265
Carter, Bram 184
cayenne 151, 177
cell synthesis 169, 200
chamomile 151, 177
chemotherapy 46, 90–91, 100, 103,
  186, 238, 258
chlorella 101, 177
cholesterol 47, 62, 96, 127, 134, 139,
  141, 146–147, 149, 151, 220, 227,
  245, 255, 265
Chronic Fatigue and Immune
  Dysfunction Association of America
  184, 289
chronic fatigue syndrome 32, 37, 52,
  122, 167, 169, 183, 191, 196, 199,
  202, 204, 217, 221, 228, 236, 255, 289
chronic pain (see pain) 3, 13, 31, 38,
  50, 57, 75, 123, 155, 159–169, 171,
  173–175, 177–179, 183, 189, 198,
  200–201, 212, 221, 229, 261, 263,
  283, 289
  use of noni with 50–51, 165–69
  Dr. Solomon's noni-user survey and
  183–85
  causes of 193–96
constipation 190, 192, 220, 233
Cooper, Russel 172–73
Cox, Paul 168
Crohn's disease 169
damnacanthal 68, 70–71, 76
depression 43, 47–48, 91, 120, 150,
  160, 163, 165, 170–171, 174,
  183–184, 188–190, 193, 198, 201–202,
  217–218, 221, 225, 231, 233, 255,
  265, 272, 283
diabetes 13, 20, 38, 43, 47–50, 52, 63,
  75, 88, 96, 105, 107–129, 134, 183,
  200, 204, 208, 218, 220, 236, 244,
  256, 260, 265–267, 269, 283, 288

use of noni with 49–50
  description of 108–120
  and "sick" cells 122
diarrhea 43, 140, 190, 192, 221, 283
diastolic 136, 144–145
Dicks, Richard 169
digestion 47–48, 90, 92, 110, 124–125,
  203, 218, 220
diverticulitis 169, 220
DL-phenylalanine 178
DMBA 85
Doell., William 9, 258
Dole 242–243, 245, 248
drug abuse 208
E. coli 35, 66–67, 213, 215, 290
elimination 90, 220
endothelial cells 64, 144
energy
  balance of 90, 92
  levels of 31, 34–35, 37–38, 91,
    94–95, 120, 140, 150, 159, 199, 202,
    231
  noni and 94–95
  restriction of 93
enzymes 55, 66, 72, 74–75, 100, 110,
  125, 140, 169, 198, 200, 208, 244
erections 63
essential oils 169, 200
estrogen 100, 171, 188
evening primrose oil 177
exercise 11, 29–30, 35, 37, 93, 95–97,
  101, 103, 111, 126, 128, 134–135,
  145, 152, 160, 165, 184, 189, 191,
  193, 264
Farden, Carl 242
fatigue 13, 32, 35, 37, 43, 52, 112, 117,
  120–122, 126, 140, 159, 167, 169,
  183–184, 186, 188–193, 196–202, 204,
  217, 221, 228–229, 232, 236, 255,
  260, 263, 289
fats 49, 99, 108–110, 124, 142, 149,

178, 289
FDA 22, 25, 57
feverfew 24–25
fiber 124, 126, 151, 220–221
fibromyalgia 37, 47, 122, 169, 183–185,
    187–198, 200–202, 212, 221, 263, 283
  causes of 188
  Dr. Solomnon's noni-user survey and
    183–85
Finland 147
foot lesions 216
fractures 43, 168–169, 219
French Polynesia 264, 270, 274, 279
Gaby, Alan 26
genitals 208
Gerson, Scott 145, 255
Gilbert R. 128
GLA 126, 177
glucose 68, 90, 109–111, 116–119, 122,
    124, 126
Golgi apparatus 71–76, 87, 129,
    142–143, 170, 173, 197–198, 200,
    212, 221
  xeronine system and 71–75
gout 18–19, 207, 221
H. pylori 21, 66, 213
Hall , Steven 9, 195, 261
Harrison, Evalee 96
Harrison, Mona 9, 95, 145, 166
Hatton, Delbert 166
headaches 24, 29, 44, 47–48, 50–51,
    140, 160, 164, 166–167, 169–170,
    184, 189–191, 202, 217–218, 221,
    226–227, 235, 259, 262, 268
heart attack 63, 133, 138, 141, 152
Heinicke, Ralph 9, 23, 37, 42, 56, 75,
    87, 170, 242, 274–275
  questionnaire of 242–52
Heinicke-Solomon Theory 71, 173
high blood pressure (see hypertension)
    3, 13, 31, 38, 43, 47–49, 63, 70, 75,

87, 96, 126–127, 131, 133–135,
    137–149, 151–153, 163, 183, 194,
    204, 207, 218, 231, 235–236, 245,
    255, 260, 265
  use of noni with 47–49, 140-46
  description of 136–141
  nitric oxide and 143–44
Hippocrates 82
Hirazumi , Anne 42, 83, 87–88, 253
hives 280
Holdman, Floyd 241
Holdman, Gayle 44
holistic healing 33
human growth hormone 63
hyperglycemia 113, 117, 120
hypericin 24
hypertension (see high blood pressure)
    38, 47, 63–64, 70, 75, 127, 133–134,
    137–139, 141, 144–146, 148, 150–153,
    283, 289
hypoglycemia 120, 165, 196
immune system 35, 38, 45, 55, 62–63,
    65–66, 75, 81, 83–84, 87–89,
    114–115, 117–118, 120–122, 129, 186,
    208, 219, 222, 228, 253, 258
  cancer and 82–84
  noni and 82–86, 213–215
  stimulation of 35
infectious arthritis 208, 221
inflammation 89, 122, 162, 168, 170,
    172, 174, 177–178, 196, 203,
    205–206, 208–212, 219, 221
injuries 36, 157, 164, 167–168, 219, 231
injury recovery 169
insomnia 163
insulin 63, 108–117, 119, 121–126,
    128–129, 257, 265
insulin-dependent diabetes 107, 112
interferon 66, 83, 88, 103, 215
interleukin 1ß 88
interleukins 88

irritable bowel syndrome 169, 190
isoflavones 100
Jim R. 114
Johns Hopkins 11, 115–116, 121
kahunas 120, 141, 165, 168, 242
Khalsa, Dharma Singh 161–62, 171, 201
kidneys 85, 113, 117, 139, 207, 210
  damage of 163
Kolodney, Samuel 9, 259
kuru 21
Levand, Oscar 67, 213
liver
  damage of 163
lungs 85, 100, 186–187, 200, 208, 210, 230
lupus 122, 159, 169, 210, 212, 257, 283
Lyons, Tommy Joe 186
M. pyrogenes 213
macrophages 43, 65–67, 83–84, 87–89
Marquesas Islands 18, 270
Marshall, Barry 21
Mayo Clinic 227–228
meditation 152, 165, 172, 238
memory loss 163, 227
menstrual cramps 57, 190, 264, 268
migraine 24, 160, 164, 166–167, 170–171, 217, 226, 235–236, 262
Mike, John 9, 215
Mike, Susan 9, 215
minerals 25, 55, 60, 72, 74–75, 99–100, 125, 169, 188, 198, 200
Morinda citrifolia 17–18, 30, 35, 41, 74
Morinda, Inc. 31, 42, 52, 253, 265, 276
morning stiffness 189–190
Morton, Julia 168, 200, 213
National Jewish Hospital 230
neck spasms 172
nerve irritation and damage 118
nervous system 161–162, 164–165, 170, 179, 201, 210, 226

neuralgia 173, 177
nitric oxide 38, 62–66, 74
  antibacterial action of 68
  cardiovascular health and 63–64
  cancer and 65
  stimulation of with noni 66–67
Nobel prize 22–23, 38, 49, 74–75, 87
noni capsules 149, 177, 279
noni juice 12, 19, 26, 31–37, 41–42, 44, 46–52, 58, 67, 70, 72, 83–85, 94–95, 102, 114, 122–123, 127–128, 140, 144, 146–148, 150–151, 157–159, 166–168, 172–176, 186–187, 194–195, 197, 199, 203–204, 209, 214–215, 217–221, 226, 229–230, 232–233, 235–236, 238, 241–246, 248–249, 253–268, 270, 273–275, 279–281, 284, 288
Non-Insulin-Dependent Diabetes 115
nono 241, 265–270, 272
norepinephrine 164
NSAIDs 163, 172
Olsen, Kelly 9, 42, 52, 253, 275
omega-3 fatty acids 24–25
osteoarthritis 169, 187, 202, 205, 211–212, 221, 258
osteoporosis 30, 96, 163
P. aeruginosa 213
pain 3, 13, 18, 24, 30–31, 35–36, 38, 47–48, 50–51, 57, 62, 75, 90, 114, 116, 122–123, 125–126, 139, 155, 158–179, 183, 185, 187–191, 194–195, 197–207, 209–212, 217–219, 221, 225–229, 231–232, 234–237, 241, 251, 255, 257, 260–261, 263, 265, 268, 283, 289
  function of 161–62
  noni and 165–69
pain gates 163–165
pain relief 50, 168, 176, 201
pancreas 63, 71, 100, 109–110, 112,

114–115, 119, 121–122, 125, 129
penis 63, 118
perfume 171
pet health 217–220, 258
phosphatidyl serine 178
physical activity 30, 35, 37–38, 82, 91,
   93, 96–97, 165, 189, 202
phytoestrogens 100
Pile, Orlando 256
polyps 227
prayer 168
prednisone 211, 230
proteins 55, 73–76, 108, 110, 169,
   197–198, 200
Proteus morganii 213
proxeroninase 57, 60, 74–75, 170, 198
proxeronine 56–61, 72–75, 87, 170,
   197–198, 212, 221, 280   history of
   56–60
Pruisiner, Stanley 21
rash 48, 163, 192, 210, 218, 229, 280,
   282
rheumatoid arthritis 88, 169, 177, 184,
   202, 208–212, 221, 231, 260, 289
rigidity 172
Riley, Carolyn 36
ringworm 213
Roger K 232
Rubiaceae 17, 290
Salmonella typhosa 67, 213
Schanely, Gloria 233–36
Schmidt's syndrome 115, 288
scopoletin 47, 55–56, 69–70, 76, 124,
   141–144, 153, 215
   high blood pressure and 70
serotonin 170–73
   chronic pain and 170–72
sex 47, 63, 96, 120
"sick" cells 38, 122
   chronic fatigue and 198
   fibromyalgia and 198

sinus infections 213
sinusitis 169, 233–234, 283
skin 17, 43, 159, 190, 192, 203–204,
   207–208, 210, 213–214, 226–227, 237,
   250, 273, 283
sleep dysfunction 170, 188, 201
soreness 159, 185, 189, 209
South Pacific 18, 241
soy isoflavones 100
St. John's wort 24, 250
Stamler, Johnathan S. 62
Staphylococcus aureus 67
steroids 159, 168, 174, 219
stiffness 30, 36, 172, 175, 177, 189–190,
   205, 209–210, 221
Story, Stephen 9, 41, 52, 245, 249, 265
stress 11, 21, 30, 37, 44, 48, 61, 101,
   125–126, 152, 160, 169, 171, 178,
   188–191, 193, 204, 207, 218, 234, 246
   reduction of 30, 101
stress headaches 169
stroke 43, 47–48, 63, 65, 107, 133,
   138–139, 141, 146, 152, 163, 218, 255
substance-P 163, 177
suicide 174
sumatriptan 171
surgery 36, 102, 158, 208, 217,
   229–230, 236, 261
survey, Dr. Solomon's noni-user 43–52
   cancer and 89–90
   diabetes and 121–22
   chronic fatigue and 183–85
   fibromyalgia and 183–85
   high blood pressure and 141–144
swelling 36, 43, 133, 167, 177, 187,
   211, 232, 251, 280
Tahiti 12, 18–19, 23, 241, 265–266,
   268–274, 279
Tahitian Noni Juice™ 31
   development of 41-42
T-cells 83, 88

tendinitis 169, 206–207, 212
The Lancet 65, 288–289
The Pain Cure 161, 165, 289
Timothy B. 123
tobacco 99
Tramel, Bill 231
Tran, Gary 167, 217, 254
tumors 63, 70, 82, 87, 100–101, 186
turmeric 177
Type I diabetes 107, 112–114, 116–117, 121, 266
Type II diabetes 50, 112, 114–120
tyramine 171
ulcers 19–21, 66, 163, 169, 213–216, 283
urinary tract 43, 208, 214
varicose veins 166, 220
vascular disorders 47
vitamins 55, 60, 72, 74–75, 99–101, 142, 169, 198, 200, 228
Wadsworth, John 9, 41, 52, 245, 249, 265

account of concerning noni 265–76
Wang, Mian-Ying 9, 51–52, 85
weight loss 113, 117, 120, 209–210, 237
Wells, John 50
wheat 98, 177
wheezing 280
white willow bark 178
Williams, Del 263
Williams, Sylvia 9, 263
wounds 19, 43, 89, 120, 169, 173, 213–214, 222
xeronine 37, 49, 55–57, 60–61, 71–76, 87, 95, 129, 142–144, 168, 170, 173, 179, 198, 200, 246, 248
xeronine system 55–56, 71, 75–76, 87, 129, 142, 168, 170, 173, 179, 200, 246
history of 56–60
Golgi apparatus and 71–75
yeast infections 192
yoga 101, 261
Zoloft 91

ABOUT THE AUTHOR

JOHNS HOPKINS CLINICALLY trained physician Neil Solomon, M.D., Ph.D., possesses an impressive list of credentials. Dr. Solomon has won numerous awards and has held various faculty professorships and appointments at some of the most prestigious universities in the country, including the Johns Hopkins School of Medicine. He was Maryland's first Secretary of Health and Mental Hygiene, has served as chair of four gubernatorial commissions, and has acted as health advisor to presidents and governors. He has appeared on television and radio talk shows, provided daily medical commentaries on CNN-TV, and for 18 years wrote a globally syndicated health advice column for the Los Angeles Times Syndicate.

Dr. Solomon is an established best-selling author (including having been on the New York Times best-selling list), and has been featured in numerous national magazines. Currently, Dr. Solomon works as a global nutritional consultant, serving corporations, nongovernment organizations of the United Nations, and the World Health Organization. Dr. Solomon is married; he and his wife have three sons.